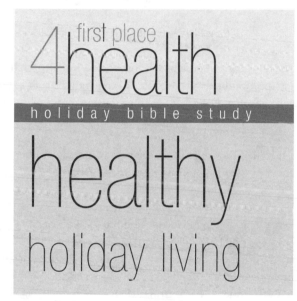

first place
4health
holiday bible study
healthy
holiday living

Published by Gospel Light
Ventura, California, U.S.A.
www.gospellight.com
Printed in the U.S.A.

Caution: The information contained in this book is intended to be solely for
informational and educational purposes. It is assumed that the First Place 4 Health
participant will consult a medical or health professional before beginning this or
any other weight-loss or physical fitness program.

Healthy holiday living.
p. cm. — (First place 4 health Bible study series)
ISBN 978-0-8307-5545-5 (trade paper)
1. Christian women—Prayers and devotions. 2. Christian women—
Health and hygiene—Prayers and devotions. 3. Thanksgiving Day—Prayers
and devotions. 4. Christmas—Prayers and devotions.
BV4844.H36 2010
242'.643—dc22
2010026422

Rights for publishing this book outside the U.S.A. or in non-English
languages are administered by Gospel Light Worldwide, an international
not-for-profit ministry. For additional information, please visit
www.glww.org, email info@glww.org, or write to Gospel Light Worldwide,
1957 Eastman Avenue, Ventura, CA 93003, U.S.A.

To order copies of this book and other Gospel Light products in bulk
quantities, please contact us at 1-800-446-7735

contents

introduction

*But seek first his kingdom and his righteousness,
and all these things will be given to you as well.*
MATTHEW 6:33

This book is not the typical First Place 4 Health Bible study. Instead, it is a special devotional tool to help you stay on course through the holidays, when many temptations will come your way. The Thanksgiving and Christmas holidays can be very busy with many social events, shopping expeditions and church activities that make it difficult to remain faithful to your commitment to living healthy. This study was written to provide order in the hectic holiday season without being a burden on your time. It will give you inspiration for each day and also challenge you to stay on course by daily applying the truths at the core of First Place 4 Health.

One Scripture verse is featured each week, and the daily devotionals use that verse as the reference. The devotionals are holiday-related and give insight and encouragement to maintain balance during the holidays. A prayer and a journaling suggestion follow each reading. A journal page has also been provided for each day to write out your prayers, thoughts and questions.

Following the six weeks of devotional readings is a section on holiday survival tips, a leader's discussion guide (for using this devotional in group settings) and menus for Thanksgiving, Christmas and New Year's Day. The Holiday Survival tips will give you valuable insights and suggestions for staying healthy spiritually, mentally, emotionally and physically through the holiday season. Recipes for additional holiday favorites are included with the menus.

At the back of this *Healthy Holiday Living* study are weekly prayer partner forms and Live It Trackers. If you are using this study in a group setting, you can fill out the weekly prayer partner form and put it into a basket during the meeting. After the meeting, you will draw out a prayer request form, and this will be your prayer partner for the week. The Live It Tracker is for you to complete at home and turn in to your leader at your weekly meeting. Remember that if you have a plan, you can remain consistent in practicing the spiritual, mental, emotional and physical disciplines you have begun in First Place 4 Health—even through the holidays!

In the following section, take a few moments to list some of your goals in each of the four core areas of your life during this holiday season and your strategies for reaching those goals.

My goals for this holiday season are:

Spiritual: _____

_____

_____

_____

_____

_____

Mental: _____

_____

_____

_____

_____

_____

Emotional: _____

_____

_____

_____

_____

_____

_____

_____

Physical: _____

_____

_____

_____

_____

_____

_____

_____

My strategies for reaching those goals are:

Spiritual: _____

_____

_____

_____

_____

_____

_____

Mental: _____

_____

_____

_____

_____

_____

_____

Emotional: _____

_____

_____

_____

_____

_____

_____

Physical: _____

_____

_____

_____

_____

_____

_____

May the next six weeks take you on a joyful journey toward complete wholeness and health! Here's to the journey!

victory in Jesus

SCRIPTURE MEMORY VERSE
*But thanks be to God! He gives us the victory through
our Lord Jesus Christ.*
1 CORINTHIANS 15:57

EVER GROWING
by Carole Lewis

Day
1

I love the song "Victory in Jesus." The words say, "He sought me and bought me with His redeeming love." I have lived the truth of this week's verse, so I can say today, "But thanks be to God! He gives *me* the victory through *my* Lord Jesus Christ."

When I joined First Place in March 1981, I didn't have a clue of how God would use this program to bring me victory in every area of my life. Back then, I was a Christian but had never given complete control of every area of my life to Christ. For some stupid reason, I thought I could handle most everything and that if I got into a jam, I would call on God.

God has used everything about this program to bring a balance to my life that I never knew was possible. When my life is balanced spiritually through a regular time spent with God in prayer and studying His Word, then I am able to reach out to others with Christ's love. Emotional balance comes as I learn that every trial "has come to pass" and that I will emerge victorious on the other side. Victory is found through Jesus living inside of me to make me more like Him.

Mental balance comes as I memorize Scripture and let the truth of God's Word play out in my life. Finally, physical balance comes as I learn to eat in a healthy way and also make exercise a regular part of my life.

My goals have changed so many times during the past 30 years of living the First Place 4 Health lifestyle, but my experience with Christ has only continued to grow as He has proven Himself faithful to me. Back in 1981, I was concerned mostly with the outward appearance—how I looked and how others perceived me.

Today, my main goal is to be able to walk upright and think clearly for as long as the Lord leaves me on this earth. Instead of caring what others think of me, I am much more concerned about what the Lord Jesus thinks of me. I want Him to be proud of me, because He is the reason that I live and breathe. When I walk into His presence, at the minute I draw my last breath on this earth, I long to hear Him say, "Well done, good and faithful servant."

I am amazed that even though I am still the same Carole who joined First Place back in 1981, I am also a new creation in all four areas of life: spiritually, emotionally, mentally and physically. I am continually being made more like my Savior, Jesus. "For those God foreknew He also predestined to be conformed to the likeness of His Son" (Romans 8:29).

Dear Lord, I am so thankful that You impressed on me to
join that First Place group in 1981, if even for
all the wrong reasons. Thank You for never giving up
on me as I have failed You and floundered
so many times. Thank You that true victory is found
in You and You alone.

Journal: Write about your most recent success in any of the four main areas of life: spirit, mind, emotions or body. Don't forget to thank God, who gives you the victory . . . and ask Him what's next.

SMALL VICTORIES, GREAT REWARD
by Carol VanAtta

So often, when I declare the victories I've experienced through Christ, I get stuck on the "big ones"—those huge nuclear wars in life where simply surviving is a victory in itself. These big victories are easy to indentify; they come to mind quickly, and they often draw an attentive crowd when revealed.

When God gives us victories such as these, it's hard not to say thank you frequently and with great fervor. After all, Christ ultimately gave us complete victory over sin and death. That's a very big deal. But what about the smaller, less obvious victories won in our daily lives?

I remember a very specific Thanksgiving Day dinner. It was rapidly turning into what I refer to as a family fiasco. The kids were bickering. The grownups were grouchy with the bickering kids. And, of course, the turkey couldn't get trimmed fast enough.

Tradition in our family has always included a special pre-dinner prayer. However, this particular year, I was wondering if we'd even eat, let alone pray together. Thankfully, a full-fledged fiasco was diverted when my mom (God bless grandmas) finished with the turkey. Everyone was eager to fill their plates with the steaming goodness and get down to the business of eating. I know I certainly was! But I also knew that if we gave into our physical hunger before satisfying our spiritual hunger, we'd be in a great deal of trouble.

"You've got to be kidding!" my son protested, his fork lifted in anticipation. "Can't we just pray later? Besides, I don't have anything big to thank Him for this year."

Normally, our family prayer time included each of us thanking God for the major victories in our lives over the past year. Right then, I realized that I had failed to teach my children something very basic but very important. Every victory is worth thanking God for. Sure, the "big ones" are awesome, but we each have little victories in Christ every single day—victories for which we often fail to thank Him.

Out of the mouths of babes, I thought, as my young daughter spoke up and said, "Thank You, God, for cupcakes and for helping me on my spelling test." Her simple thank-you was all we needed to start celebrating and thanking God for our victories. I knew then that we would make it through Thanksgiving with attitudes filled with gratitude, not grumpiness.

As I brought that heartfelt prayer to a close, I was able to thank God for the victory we had just enjoyed while sitting around the table—a special victory for a very special day.

Thanksgiving is the perfect holiday to honor God for the victories He has orchestrated in our lives. Why not start a new tradition and thank God for making you victorious through Him? And remember to celebrate the many battles won (big and small) along the way.

Father, so often I forget to thank You for who You are, and that it is You who gives me the victory in every area of life. Thanks for providing all that I need, and much more, according to Your riches in glory.

Journal: Every day for the next week, record what you are thankful for, no matter how seemingly insignificant. At the end of seven days, reread those pages and reflect on how richly God has blessed you.

SWEET SUCCESS

by Delilah Dirksen

Just after Thanksgiving a couple of years ago, I heard a news story about the average American gaining seven pounds over the holiday season. Whether true or not, the potential weight gain was enough to motivate me to beat the odds. Understanding the importance of accountability, I was thankful to have joined the First Place 4 Health holiday session at my church.

Class leader Beth Johnson and I discovered that we both were considering giving up sugar for the holidays. Sugar had never been a draw for me until I married into a wonderful family with a contagious appreciation for sweets. The temptation was ever present.

Beth and I committed to a "sugar pact." This was to be a birthday gift to Jesus. After all, this seemed so insignificant compared to the sacrifice He made for us. Believing that God would provide us with the strength, we agreed to no white sugar and no desserts, and to pray for each other.

There were many victories. One night my husband placed our son's leftover birthday cake on the table for dessert. I redirected my attention to the dishes in the sink. Having recently spoken with Beth about this cake, our sugar pact was at the top of my thoughts—but so was that cake! I thought, *Maybe just a sliver . . .*

I dried my soapy hands and marched back toward the table with fork in hand. Instead of going right for the cake, I hesitated and circled the table like a bird of prey while proclaiming a First Place 4 Health Scripture memory verse: "No temptation has seized you except what is common to man. And God is faithful; he will not let you be tempted beyond what you can bear. But when you are tempted, he will also provide a way out so that you can stand up under it" (1 Corinthians 10:13)!

While this was going on, our nine-year-old lunged out of his chair and grabbed the First Place 4 Health "It's Not in Here" magnet off the refrigerator. He scurried back to his seat and flashed the magnet at me over the cake. We all laughed, and my craving was instantly conquered. Gospel artist Mandisa's lyrics, "With You by my side, I am victorious," describe how I felt.

This set out to be a gift to Jesus, but *I* felt like I received the gift. The victory was so sweet, I continued to deny myself sugar for the entire year. I broke a five-year plateau, lost 14 pounds and felt closer to God as a result of my experience. The sugar was replaced with healthier choices, while cravings for other foods dissipated. Beth also lost weight and achieved her health goals, and others even started making "sugar pacts"!

Is your kitchen's "sweetness" sabotaging your health goals? I am not necessarily recommending you do a sugar pact, but whatever your challenge is this season, turn to the One whose birthday we prepare to celebrate—as there is nothing sweeter than feeling the victory from He who gives us the strength within.

Father, because You have saved me not only from the penalty of sin but from the power of sin, I know that I can resist all the "sweet" things in life that are nothing more than Satan's attempts to harm me and turn my feet from the path to health. Thank You for giving me the strength to do what I know is best for me.

Journal: Sugar is an enemy, but it's not the only enemy to achieving your health goals. Take inventory and see if you've been flirting with a harmful thought or action. Write about it, and remind yourself "it's not in here!"

WHAT THE MIND CANNOT CONCEIVE
by Karrie Smyth

What a precious promise! God gives us victory through our Lord Jesus Christ! When I began the First Place 4 Health program in 2002, I never could have guessed the victory God had in store for me as I learned to give Christ first place. I was drawn by Carole's testimony of balance even during the hardest seasons of life. God used her testimony to give me the faith to believe that He could do it for me. As I learned to seek first His kingdom and His righteousness, I began to walk a life of balance. For those of you battling chaos, He gives us the victory through Jesus Christ!

As months passed, I came to realize the victory that God gives when we honor Him with our bodies. I lost the weight that I had struggled with for years, and God began defeating the idol of food that had held such power over me. If you are battling the idolatry of food, God gives the victory through our Lord Jesus Christ!

When my father lost his battle with cancer, and grief threatened to make me lose my way, God didn't let go of me. When I was faithless, He remained faithful to me. If you are battling the grief of a seemingly insurmountable loss, God gives the victory through our Lord Jesus Christ!

In 2007, the Lord challenged me to ask Him for healing from the ravages of Crohn's disease. I had to confess my unbelief. When we are willing to cry out, "I do believe; help me overcome my unbelief!" (Mark 9:24), we find that God gives victory through our Lord Jesus Christ! Thanks be to God that He saw fit to heal me and there is not even a trace of Crohn's disease left in my body!

Without a doubt, the greatest victory that God has given me in the last eight years has been the absolutely miraculous healing in my marriage. The victory that God has won there defies words! Eight years ago, I thought that the victory was measurable on the scales. I am so thankful that that was only the beginning!

What about you? Is your heart overflowing with thanksgiving to God, or are there some things that are battling against your grateful heart? Give the Lord your battles. Give God your thanks. He will give you the victory through our Lord Jesus Christ.

Father, You overwhelm me with Your love demonstrated through Your power to give me the victory even when I am thinking that life will never be good again. You always do so much more than I could ever ask for.

Journal: Is there something in your life that is gaining ground in the battle against your grateful heart? God has already won the victory, so start thanking Him for what He's already done and won, even in the midst of your battle.

YOU GAIN MORE THAN YOU LOSE
by Paulette McDonald

When I started First Place 4 Health, I had selfish motives. It was all about losing weight. It didn't take long for the scales to be removed from my eyes in this area. Seeing God for who He is and knowing what Jesus did to His physical body to save me, and what I was doing to my own body to hurt me, was truly a divine moment.

I am thankful to have encountered God in such a way that my heart was not only softened, but reality became truth. Questions began to come into my mind: *If my intentions are truly to serve the Lord, then how am I able to do this without my health and my body? Do I really fear the Lord if I continue to treat my body this way? How can anyone in the world receive what I am saying about Jesus if I cannot even take care of myself?*

When you begin to focus on your health, you become mindful of the food you eat, and weight loss becomes a reality. But true accomplishment comes when you have a change in your heart about your body as the temple the Lord gave you. Just as there has to be a change in your heart for you to decide to follow Christ, there has to be a change in your heart to begin taking care of your body and allow the Lord to be victorious in this area.

Every day my children show me something they have done—a bug they've caught or a new funny face they have learned or a beautiful finger painting on their bedroom wall. And they respond to my praise. I've come to realize that every day I need to be renewed by gratitude for all that God has done and praise Him. I am thankful for the Lord showing me that the ladies in our group not only serve a purpose of accountability, but also in renewing me from the terrible life of overeating I was rescued from.

I have rediscovered the praise God deserves. For even in my disobedience, He is still able to use me. Even though I could recite the fruit of the Spirit and forget that self-control was one of them, He was still patient with my slow learning. Victory begins by giving thanks to God.

Father, thank You for never giving up on me and for guiding me to a health plan that puts You first above all things. Thank You for showing me the importance of praising You who are supreme above all.

Journal: How has my health goal changed from being all about me to being more about what God is doing in me?

NO LONGER BATTLE WEARY
by Sarah Mielke

Thanksgiving has always been one of my favorite times of the year. With this holiday comes the sights and smells from my childhood days. I remember my aunt's homemade broccoli casserole (with lots of cheese, so even the kids would eat broccoli!), a table set with my grandmother's finest china and, of course, hot homemade bread! We would watch the Macy's Thanksgiving Day parade and spend the rest of the day together as a family, eating and napping.

Memories of holidays are usually surrounded by food. When you mention "Thanksgiving," we always muster up an image of a well-set table, golden brown turkey and all the trimmings. Over the past few years, my focus has been drawn away from the food and toward my family. Since I have been following First Place 4 Health principles, the way I approach these times of feast has also changed. I realize that I cannot have victory in Christ without some sort of battle. Victory cannot come by any other means than a battle. I come to the Thanksgiving table with the expectation of temptation and the tools with which I have learned to fight it.

My battle lies in food. I have come to realize that my choices dictate what I eat. No thing (food included!) has a hold on me that Christ has not given me the power to overcome. No longer does food hold me captive. It is my choice to eat specific, delicious holiday foods. It is my choice as to how much of them to have. And, I know when I leave the Thanksgiving table this year, I am reminded that God gives the victory to me through Jesus: victory in my salvation, victory in my battle with food, victory in everyday life. I am most thankful for that.

*Father, thank You that through Jesus, nothing is destined to enslave me—
including my food choices during the holidays. You have given me the weapons
I need to resist temptation and enjoy Thanksgiving with my family.*

Journal: What will be different this Thanksgiving as you participate in a tradition built around delicious food? Be specific about the weapons at your command.

Day 7

A GIFT THAT LASTS
by Vicki Heath

If your children are like ours (actually, if you are like me), then you understand that children can lose hours and hours of sleep anticipating THE event—opening their Christmas presents. Sometimes the gifts actually match up to the anticipation. With maturity, we learn that giving Christmas gifts is simply following the pattern from God's gift "wrapped in swaddling clothes and lying in a manger." Thanks be to God because "He gives." That is His nature. He gave us the ultimate gift of His love in the victory of eternal life through Jesus Christ. Knowing that God's grace in Jesus Christ is an "indescribable gift," we can use gift-giving to share Jesus with others. Here are a few ideas.

1. Make a list of people who do not know Christ but know you well enough to accept a gift from you. Select two people and bless them with an inexpensive but thoughtful gift.

2. Consider the unique interests of each person and what each needs to learn about Jesus. Ask the Holy Spirit to reveal to you gifts that match both your friends' interests and their need to learn about Christ.

3. Wait for the Spirit to guide you to His innovative solution to your request.

The gift could be a Christian book, a CD or a picture. Or the gift could be yourself: a round of golf, a visit to a park, or some other activity to be shared. While you spend time together, the Lord will create opportunities for you to share about Christ . . . and then give thanks. After all, isn't that what Christ did? He gave us Himself. "Thanks be to God for His indescribable gift!" and "Thanks be to God. He gives us the victory through our Lord Jesus Christ." He gives, and we are thankful people.

Father, thank You for the indescribable gift of Yourself. I am overwhelmed with Your love. The only acceptable and worthy response is to give You my heart, without reservation. My hope is in You.

Journal: Record the names of two people you know who need the Lord. Ask the Holy Spirit to reveal a gift for each that would create an opportunity to talk to them about the gift of Jesus, and write this in the space below.

Group Prayer Requests

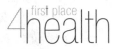

Today's Date: _____

Name	Request

Results

_____
_____
_____
_____
_____
_____

no
worries

SCRIPTURE MEMORY VERSE

*Do not be anxious about anything, but in everything, by prayer and petition
with thanksgiving, present your requests to God.*

PHILIPPIANS 4:6

ASK IN MY NAME
by Carole Lewis

Day
1

As I write these words, we have two grandchildren, Christen and Tal, who are taking their final exams and will graduate from college within the next two weeks. This morning, I received a Facebook message from Christen saying that she was going through finals all this week. How wonderful to be able to assure her that we are all praying for them to do well on their finals and to graduate.

Sometimes, when I feel anxious, it is hard for me to pray effectively. This is especially true when someone I love is going through a tough time. My husband, Johnny, is two-thirds of the way through 15 chemo treatments, and this is an anxious time for me. Will the chemo kill good cells along with the bad ones? Will his immune system stay strong enough to fight infection?

During such times, it is really important to ask others to pray for us. The Bible tells us in Romans 8:26 that the Holy Spirit prays for us when we don't know how to pray. I believe that one of the greatest blessings of First Place 4 Health is that we have the privilege to pray for each other.

A woman in my First Place 4 Health class shared with me yesterday that she received a job offer this week after being out of work for several months. She wrote her need for work on her prayer request last week. She works out of her home as a technical writer, and this job is big and has the potential to last for at least a year.

God hears our prayers and knows the deepest desires of our heart even when we don't know how to pray. Sometimes when I feel anxious, I just say to God, "You know," because He does know, and He cares about me and my needs.

What do you feel anxious about right now? Is it a health issue? Finances? Your weight? Your marriage? Your children? Jesus knows your every need, and He cares about your situation. He does His best work when we don't know how to pray. Ask a trusted friend or a member of your First Place 4 Health class to pray for you during this time. The Holy Spirit is already praying for you, and the Bible says, "Where two or three come together in my name, there am I with them" (Matthew 18:20). Also, Ecclesiastes 4:12 says, "A cord of three strands is not quickly broken."

There is power in prayer. I believe that the reason my husband, who has stage 4 prostate cancer, is still alive after 12 years is because of the prayers of people all over the world on his behalf. Don't be afraid to ask others to pray for you. This is the greatest benefit of being in the family of God.

Dear Lord, thank You for the blessing of
being Your child. Thank You for the brothers and sisters I have
because I am part of Your family. Help me to ask for
prayer when I need it and to be faithful to pray when
others ask me to pray for them.

Journal: What are you more likely to do—worry or pray? Record a problem you're facing today and also write the name of a close friend or group of friends you will ask to pray for you. Then ask!

MY BURDEN IS LIGHT
by David Self

I've been anxious about worry for most of my life. The best I can fig-ure, my sanguine nature (Lighten up!) wars with my spiritual gift of administration (Is it safe? Is it economical? Will it work?). The result-ing combination produced an honor roll student who worried about every test. Classes were more of a challenge to excel than an opportu-nity to learn.

So, when I enrolled in First Place 4 Health, the class and its expec-tations were not without stress. Change the way I eat? Exercise every day? (And worst of all . . .) Record my weight every week? I have to say that I went home and had a long talk with the Lord. I told Him that I didn't need more stress in my life. And whose business was it anyway re-garding the way I planned meals? And, to tell you the truth, I wasn't sure I wanted to keep track of my meals, my weight and exercise regu-larly. I read through the first Bible study and reviewed the class com-mitment and then fumed a little more.

And then, God seemed to bring Philippians 4:6 to my mind. As Kenneth Taylor paraphrases the first part of the verse, "Do not be anx-ious about anything but in everything, by prayer and petition, with thanksgiving, present your requests to God." So, I prayed the commit-ment back to God. I said, "Dear Lord, if this ministry is for me, I need Your strength and good favor. Help me not to worry about things I can't control, and focus on the things I can. Give me the ability to have fun in the class and really learn about this temple You've given me. And I thank You in advance for the blessings I will receive."

And I did (have fun, that is). At the end of the course, my First Place 4 Health teacher joked that I was the only student he's ever had who lost weight and had pizza once a week. I even had some turkey, dress-ing and giblet gravy on Thanksgiving. I found that daily exercise became less of a chore and more of a stress reliever. As I lost weight and got into shape, I felt better and worried less.

The prayer of surrender took the stress off me and appropriated God's strength. As you thank God this season for His many blessings, don't fail to take advantage of His prescription for stress-free living.

Remember: when you're worrying, you're not praying. And, when you're praying, it's almost impossible to worry.

Father, help me stop worrying about things I can't control, and help me focus on the things I can. Thank You in advance for giving me Your peace and contentment in whatever circumstances I encounter.

Journal: Are you a natural worrier? Write a prayer that expresses your trust in God's ability to carry your mental load, and then, to the best of your ability, rest from your burden.

GOT PEACE?
by Karrie Smyth

Day **3**

Life offers us no shortage of things that tempt us with anxiety. The pressures of jobs, relationships, parenting, keeping house, paying bills, eating healthy . . . even balancing all of the above can produce an abundance of anxiety—if you let them. The apostle Paul, under the direction of the Holy Spirit, wrote, "Do not be anxious" (Philippians 4:6). When I realized this meant that I actually had a choice of whether or not to give in to anxiety, my life started changing for the better.

You see, when the Lord gives us a command, like this one, He always provides how to do it. When we recognize the familiar feeling of anxiety, we are to stop and take our feelings and concerns to the Lord in prayer. Not only that, but we are to do so with thanksgiving.

No matter how ominous the circumstance, we can always begin by thanking the Lord that we don't have to face it alone. Thank the Lord that He is able to do infinitely more than we could ask or dream and He is working all things—truly *all* things—together for our good, whether it feels that way or not. Thank Him that nothing is impossible for Him. As you pray and express your gratitude to the Lord, it will become much easier to present your requests to God and then leave them there with Him. When we begin to thank God for what He has done for us in the past and what He desires to do in and through us in the future, our gratitude will grow and our eyes will begin to look above our problems into the face of our God. That's when the most awesome thing happens: peace replaces anxiety!

You see, this verse is an instruction that is followed by a promise: "And the peace of God, which transcends all understanding, will guard your hearts and your minds in Christ Jesus" (Philippians 4:7). How awesome! How amazing! How like God's economy! He lifts my anxiety and guards me with His peace.

Let's not allow anxiety to color our lives this holiday season. It's not necessary. It is avoidable. We have so many things to be thankful for. Let's develop an *attitude of gratitude*. When the things of the world press in on us, let's consciously count our blessings and express our thanks to the Lord. Let's present our requests to Him and leave them to Him to handle in His time and in His way; and then let's receive His peace. It transcends our circumstances. Thank You, Lord!

*Father, Your Word tells me that I have a choice when
circumstances seem to be against me. I choose to obey Your command
to thank You for the circumstance and receive Your peace . . .
help me make that choice every time.*

Journal: Record your top concern and rephrase it with words of gratitude for what God does in working in and through you for His good purposes. Whatever the outcome, don't forget to thank Him for His peace that passes all human understanding.

WALKING THE PEACE PATH
by Martha Rogers

In late October 1999, I underwent my second mastectomy. Five years had elapsed between the first one and the mammogram that discovered this tumor. I thought perhaps I had defeated cancer, but that was not to be. This verse in Philippians, which I memorized in First Place 4 Health, became my verse for getting through this second trial.

Since God had brought me through before, I could trust Him to do the same this time. Being thankful for cancer is not easy, but it was easy to be thankful for everything He had done in those five years. Concentrating on the good and being thankful will put the present dilemma in the proper perspective.

Crisis comes and goes in our lives like the ebb and flow of the tide. Whether we're ready for each crisis or not depends on our trust and faith in our heavenly Father. After all, He knew the days of our lives before we were even born. He knows every hair on our head, and He knows every sorrow we bear. When we are anxious about things in our lives, and we worry about them, we are telling God that we don't have complete trust. Let God be in control; turn the problems over to Him, and He will keep His promises.

One of those promises is to supply our every need. Sometimes we may not agree with how He accomplishes that, but we can be sure that He will not fail us.

The first Thanksgiving after that second surgery was blessed, indeed, because the doctor informed me that he had removed all of the cancer and no lymph nodes were involved. In addition, he was not recommending any radiation or chemo. He said he'd see me in six months for a check-up, and that was it.

What a great cause for giving thanks and praising God that holiday season! Every Thanksgiving, my family remembers that time, and once again we praise God and rejoice for the years He has given us to be together.

No matter how dark, scary or horrible a situation may be, letting go and letting God be in control is the true path to peace. The verse following Philippians 4:6 tells us that when we do present our requests to God with thanksgiving, we will have the peace that transcends all understanding.

When worry and fear threaten to come in and quench the Holy Spirit, we must remember this verse and seek the peace that only He can bring. This holiday season, thank God for whatever your circumstances are, because nothing is too big for our God to handle, and your circumstances are no surprise to Him. He is already working out the solution before you even ask. Trust in the Lord with all your heart, and He will guide you in the way you should go.

Father, when I am overwhelmed by fear and dread, I know
that You are already guiding me to the path that is Your perfect peace.
Praise Your glorious name!

Journal: Tell God about a chronic fear or anxiety You want Him to carry for you.

MORE THAN WE COULD ASK FOR

by P. J. Bahr

For years, I prayed that God would bring someone into my life to do a Bible study with me on weight loss. My weight had escalated after I married—not drastically, but enough that I knew I had begun carrying an extra and unnecessary 20 pounds, and I was afraid there was no end in sight if left to my own devices. I believed that if I could just do a Bible study on weight loss, with a friend, it would be the key to success in losing my weight and keeping it off permanently.

After more than three years of praying that specific prayer, God just wasn't answering me. I couldn't figure out why He wouldn't bring someone into my life to do this with me. There were so many days I was tremendously discouraged and impatient. Out of desperation, I'd seek out a girlfriend, a coworker, a relative or anyone, but I was always met with rejection. Sometimes a girlfriend would say, "Sure!" and then not follow through on meeting together. Other times, I seemed to be just expecting God to drop someone on my front porch to say, "Okay! Here I am! Let's do this together!"

Then, in 2004, I stood as the teacher at the front of my very first class of "Giving Christ First Place." Looking out over the 30-plus people, I began to cry and said, "I prayed for God to bring me someone to do a Bible study with me on weight loss. He didn't bring just one person; He brought me more than 30 people!"

God has done immeasurably more than I could ever ask or imagine through First Place 4 Health. He has taught me balance in all four areas of my life: my emotions, my body, my mind and my spirit. He has proven the words of Philippians 2:13 that "it is God who works in you to will and to act according to his good purpose." His timing—His purpose, not mine.

When you feel that God isn't answering your prayers, or isn't showing you any signs at all that He is even hearing you, don't be anxious, but continue persevering in prayer. He may be working behind the scenes to answer your prayer above and beyond all that you could ever ask or imagine. Then you will be blessed to say, as I have, "I thank God that He has given me the victory through my Lord Jesus Christ!"

"Because of the LORD's great love we are not consumed, for his compassions never fail. They are new every morning; great is your faithfulness" (Lamentations 3:22-23). Remember these words. God's power is sure and His promises are true.

Father, when I don't ask for the right things, or when I get impatient for
Your answer, help me desire only You, and not what You can do.

Journal: What are you asking God for that He hasn't answered yet? Stop focusing on what you want and start asking God for what He wants. Record the changes in your attitude and your request.

GOD-CENTERED THANKS
by Sherry Mazza

For most of my thirties, I was gripped by serious anxiety. Self-focus on how I was feeling kept me from enjoying life; my peace and contentment were not evident to anyone around me. Even though I loved the Lord, for many years I could not gain victory in this area of fear and worry.

I started First Place 4 Health five years ago, and the members of my group began praying for me. The Lord began to turn things around when I was doing one of the First Place 4 Health Bible studies. It encouraged us to write five things in the morning and five things in the evening for which we were thankful. If you did that for one month, you would be grateful for 300 things! How would I do that? I was not happy or grateful for anything. So I started with the basics. For example, "I am happy the sun came up this morning," "I am happy the birds are singing," and so forth. This began my habit of writing in a prayer journal.

At first it was difficult, but with the encouragement of my First Place 4 Health group, I continued day after day; my focus became less self-centered and more God-centered. I began to see all the wonderful things the Lord has done for me.

Through journaling, my focus improved and my anxiety became less and less, my joy has been restored and I have learned to cast my cares on Him and trust Him with the outcome.

Any time I become anxious, I bring it to the Lord and thank Him in advance for the good plan He has for me. Are you anxious and cast down? Do you have an attitude of gratitude? This holiday season, try keeping a gratitude journal and see all the wonderful things the Lord has done for you.

"And the peace of God, which transcends all understanding, will guard your hearts and your minds in Christ Jesus" (Philippians 4:7). The Lord doesn't want you to be anxious this holiday season. If you practice combating anxiety with gratitude toward God, you will be amazed at the result it will produce in your spirit.

Father, help me show Your peace and contentment to people I meet
so they will notice the difference and You will be glorified.

Journal: Record five things, both morning and evening, for which you are thankful. Keep it up and you'll be amazed at your new focus and what a little thankfulness can do.

_____

_____

_____

_____

_____

_____

_____

_____

_____

_____

_____

_____

_____

_____

_____

_____

_____

_____

ANY BASKET WILL DO!
by Vicki Heath

If your family is like ours, you probably start receiving Christmas cards right after Thanksgiving. Though I love receiving them, I am always in a quandary over what to do with them. I love hearing from my friends and cannot bear the thought of throwing them away! We have tried hanging them up around the fireplace, which proved not to be so safe. We have tried taping them around the doorway of the kitchen—quite annoying, the tape never holds. We have tried putting them on the refrigerator, but eventually run out of magnets and they fall off and scatter everywhere when you open the door! Finally, I started putting them in a big basket on the kitchen table.

One morning, my daughter, Megan, pulled one out, noticed who it was from and the sweet family picture and said, "Mommy, can we pray for the Kellers?" That was the beginning of our "thankful prayers for our friends" Christmas card tradition! When they start arriving, we place them in a basket on the table—any basket will do! At mealtime, one of our children chooses a card from the basket, and we pray for that family. We thank God for their friendship and ask Him to supply all of their needs in Christ Jesus this coming year. It has been a wonderful reminder that we should be grateful for the abundance of friends God has brought into our lives over the years, some quite forgotten!

"Pray in the Spirit on all occasions with all kinds of prayers and requests. With this in mind, be alert and always keep on praying for all the saints" (Ephesians 6:18).

Father, You created us for relationship with You.
Help me desire more of You. And help me appreciate all
those You have given me to love.

Journal: You may want to establish your own "thankful prayers for friends" Christmas card tradition. Or ask God what else you and your family could do to honor the relationships He has given you.

Group Prayer Requests

first place
4health

Today's Date: _____

Name	Request

Results

_____
_____
_____
_____
_____
_____

name above
every name

Scripture Memory Verse
*You will be with child and will give birth to a son,
and you are to give him the name Jesus.*

Luke 1:31

HONORING THE FAMILY NAME
by Carole Lewis

Day
1

When our son, John, was born, I wanted to name him John Talton Lewis Jr., after his daddy. His daddy had always gone by "Johnny," so we decided to call our little boy John. When John grew up and married Lisa, their first child was a boy, and they named him John Talton Lewis, III, and called him Tal to differentiate between Johnny and John.

Have you ever thought about the fact that God the Father chose the name for His only Son, Jesus? The angel was only a messenger delivering the news from God to Mary.

Names are as important today as they were at the time Jesus was born. I knew a little boy named Dan McGrew who spent his childhood struggling to overcome the negative connotation of his name.

As believers, we have been adopted into the family of God because of the sacrifice Jesus made when He died on the cross at Calvary. There never will be a name quite as special as the name Jesus.

The Christmas season is a time when the world's eyes and ears are open to the name of Jesus. Christmas carols play in the shopping malls, and cards, wrapping paper and gifts point to the "reason for the season."

This year, let's think of ways we can bring honor to our "family name" of Jesus. Here are a few things we could do:

- Bring joy to someone in a nursing home by giving him or her the gift of time.

- Take your kids to deliver gifts to a family who needs them.

- Invite a lost friend or someone who is lonely to go with you to a Christmas celebration at church.

- Invite a single friend or someone who would spend Christmas alone to spend Christmas with your family.

- Encourage your family to each give an amount to world missions that is greater than they spend on any single gift for each other.

- Show Christ's love to every cashier you encounter this season.

- Write a note to someone in your life who has impacted your Christian growth.

The crass commercialism of Christmas can be used as a time for those of us in the family of God to make a real difference in our world. Will we do it?

*Dear Lord, I pray that this Christmas season will find
me showing Your love to everyone I meet. Show me ways to impact
my world by bringing honor to Your precious name. Thank You for
adopting me into Your family. In Jesus' name, Amen.*

Journal: What specific things do you plan to do this Christmas season to bring honor to the name of Jesus?

LIVING IN THE MIRACLE
by Barb Lukies

Can you just imagine what it would have been like for Mary, probably only 14 years old, and a virgin, being told that she would give birth to a Son and He would be called Jesus, the Savior of the world? Imagine Joseph's reaction, knowing that he had not fathered the child.

It's an understatement to say that Mary's unplanned pregnancy would have been frowned on back in those days, let alone her trying to convince others it was a miraculous conception. She was still a virgin and betrothed to Joseph in a Jewish marriage. How would you respond to being told that news? Just imagine how your daughter would try to explain that event to you today. What would your family's reaction be?

Today there are many single teenage girls with babies, and many un-wed couples having babies. But to also have to explain how the conception took place would qualify you for psychiatric therapy: "Well, let's see! I had a vision from the Holy Spirit who told me I would conceive a son and call him Jesus; and even though I am a virgin, I am going to have a baby."

Then to realize that this child wasn't just an average child, but He would save the world and bring life to many. He would be a scholar at a young age, perform miracles, heal the sick and help the poor and needy, the widow, the isolated and marginalized. He would later pay the ulti-mate sacrifice for our sins and die at the age of only 33, after serving three years in ministry so that thousands upon thousands of people could live eternally. What a scary yet awesome privilege it would have been to be handpicked by God to birth His only Son.

As we reflect on this verse, what are some of the miracles that God has done in your life that you weren't prepared for? Take some time to plan a celebration of Christ's birth this year with understanding of and devotion for the true meaning of Christmas. Who can you share Christ's message with this year?

Lord Jesus, I don't understand the miracle of
"God with us," but I praise You with all my heart that I can live
in the miracle of Your salvation every day.

Journal: How are you going to celebrate the birth of Jesus this Christmas to be a testimony to others and bring Him glory?

HAPPY BIRTHDAY, JESUS!
by Betha McGee

I enjoy birthday celebrations, especially the birthdays of others! History tells us that the Egyptians were among the first to celebrate birthdays, around 3000 B.C., but you had to be the queen or a male member of royalty. Later, the Greeks began the celebration—with cake and candles—but only for the men folk, and they continued celebrating that birthday long after the man had died—much as we do George Washington's birthday. The country folk of Germany started the tradition of celebrating everyone's birthday, considering the children's to be the most important. Makes me even prouder to know some of my ancestors came from Germany!

Someone in my family or group of friends is likely to get a call or email from me the day before their big day. I remind them to celebrate that day—it is the last day in their life that they will be that age again!—*then* celebrate the next day, the first day of their new year! After all, why not celebrate two days? Too often we do not celebrate the good things in life. Another year sure beats the alternative!

The best birthday to celebrate is the birth of our Savior! Getting the house decorated—putting out the manger scene—filling the house with aroma from the kitchen and the sounds of Christmas carols only adds to the celebration. On Christmas Eve, take time to read the Christmas story and talk about baby Jesus.

I enjoy making candy molds of the manger with baby Jesus, Mary and Joseph, putting them on top of a cake and then placing some of the animals, shepherds and wise men on the sides. If I have time to make the cake, all the better; but a Bundt cake or angel food cake serves the purpose. If the manger scene is white chocolate, then we use a milk chocolate icing, and vice versa. When possible, it is fun to let the children decorate the cake. Place candles on the top for everyone present.

Then all sing "Happy Birthday" to Jesus on Christmas day. If no children are present, do it anyway. I have even done it alone and then given the cake away to neighbors.

Last year was the first Christmas my new husband and I spent together, and we were going out of town. I made the candy molds and bought cakes and frosting for each family member who lived near us. We then took the same thing to the families we would be seeing at our destination. I probably had more fun than anyone, but to me, celebrating the birth of Christ is an important event, and one I enjoy sharing. Christmas is more than giving and receiving gifts; it is thanking God for His Son He named Jesus.

Father, help me to be grateful and excited about
my life and mindful of Your purposes for me. Thank You
for my new birth in Jesus Christ.

Journal: Plan a "Happy Birthday, Jesus" party for your children, or for neighborhood children—complete with activities, singing, gifts and a reminder that Jesus' birth is God's gift to us.

WHAT'S IN A NAME?
by Betha McGee

Day **4**

As a young newlywed, I was devastated to be told that if I should ever become pregnant, I would probably not be able to carry the child. It was not long until I knew the heartbreak of that prophecy! A couple of years went by, and I again was told that we were going to have a child. I often thought about Mary, the mother of Jesus, and how she was told not only that she would have a Son, but that the child would be named Jesus. We finally settled on a name for a boy and for a girl. You see, this was before the newfangled ultrasound that could tell you the gender of your baby.

The time came for our baby to be delivered, and when I woke, I was told we had a son! We named him Bill Douglas. Because of the doctor's concern for having another child of our own, we were discussing adoption when we found out we were expecting again! We already had a girl's name picked out but had difficulty agreeing on a boy's name. I again thought of Mary, who already had her name for her baby!

While I spent most of my pregnancy in bed, I studied the life of David, a man after God's own heart. Our second child came early, and we named him David Alan. We were told that we should wait until David started to school if we wanted another child. We did not heed that advice.

This time we changed the girl's name. We tried to settle on a boy's and came up with Stephen Paul. This child came prematurely. And she was so small! Her name was on the birth certificate before I woke up. It was not the name we had discussed! Her dad named her Barbara and I added Lynn.

I again thought of Mary and how God took care of the name for her. As proud of our children as we could be, I knew that my husband and I would have to work hard to bring up our children so they would want to follow Christ. We made our mistakes, and I often felt kinship to Mary when the Bible said, "Mary treasured up all these things and pondered them in her heart" (Luke 2:19).

We are grateful to God for the children He gave us and for the adults that they have become. We were more grateful that through Mary, God loved us so much that He gave us His only begotten Son (see John 3:16)!

Father, thank You for sending us Your only begotten Son, Jesus, the name that is above every name; the name at which every knee shall bow and every tongue confess that Jesus Christ is Lord, to the glory of God the Father (see Philippians 2:9-10).

Journal: Research the names of Jesus found in the Old and New Testaments ("prince of peace," "bread of life," "I am"). Whenever you forget who it is that was born as a tiny baby to be your Savior, go through that list and wonder anew at what God did.

Day
5

WORTH THE WAIT
by Judy Marshall

The familiar story goes on to tell us that Mary answered, "May it be to me as you have said" (Luke 1:38). As God's children, we who celebrate Christ's birth know how wonderful these words were. Jesus would be born to die as our sacrifice and then resurrected from death to give us eternal life. I wonder when it was that Mary understood all the adjustments she would make for God's miracle.

Unlike Mary, we might protest, "Nine months is a really long time. I'll have to leave the comforts of home. I'm being asked to do something too difficult. What if . . .? How . . .? What about . . .? Yes, but . . . why?" These thoughts and questions also may be part of our "familiar story" in the First Place 4 Health journey. Can we adjust for God's miracle?

"This diet is too long!" On Day One, the wait is a slow 270-something days. But as we're faithful to one meal at a time, and the 270-plus days have finally passed, we discover it's been a mere nine months. Patience is rarely easy, but great results diligently planned are well worth the wait!

"Leave comforts? No way!" Comforts come wrapped in different packages. One may look like leaving the fast-food lane to learn to plan and prepare healthy meals and snacks. Another looks like setting the alarm 20 minutes early to make time to prepare our hearts and our day with Bible study. Yet another looks like deciding to give up watching a sitcom to take a walk with family. It could be high-calorie comfort food exchanged for nutritious choices to fuel our bodies. Ahh! These new habits can be rewarding and comforting!

"First Place 4 Health is just too hard during holidays." Do you agree that it's more difficult to follow the Spirit's leading than to fall in line behind yourself? I used to love taking myself to bountiful buffets and dessert bars. But I've found that when He leads me in discipline and self-control, I'm able to walk away from out-of-control eating and mindless

choices I later regret. During holidays my daily habits are: (1) Recite Deuteronomy 30:11: "Now what I am commanding you today is not too difficult for you or beyond your reach"; and (2) pray for God's help when I'm tempted by decadent choices during these festive seasons.

The familiar-story questions we ask, if allowed in our thinking, make it difficult to stay focused on our desire for wholeness and balance. However, if we call them by their real name, WHINING, we can turn them loose to make room for "whatever" thoughts listed in Philippians 4:8, and to encouraging others.

In the Christmas story, Matthew says, "They will call him Immanuel . . . God with us" (Matthew 1:23) to fulfill the prophecy of Isaiah. What a wonderful gift all year long! God with us—even in our journey toward good health! Let's accept God's gift and the First Place 4 Health challenge with Mary's words of surrender: "May it be to me as you have said."

Father, I surrender my whining about how hard it
is to keep walking the path toward balanced health. As I make
choices for my health this holiday season, may I show You the
same acceptance Mary offered.

Journal: What thoughts are counterproductive to your making wise choices every day, and especially during the holidays? What is the next right step for you?

LIKE YOUR FATHER
by June Chapko

Day
6

I often wondered what my mother was thinking when she chose my name back in the mid-forties. Babies born during that era came out with basic "no frills" monikers. Many were named after relatives, but essentially the common names were simple, like Mary, Carol, Betty, and my own name, June.

Given the fact that I was born just four days before Christmas, it may well have been that my mother was wishing it were the month of June rather than the blizzard conditions of December. My parents never revealed how they decided on my name, but I have often wondered what it means. I've enjoyed a couple benefits from its simplicity: it's easy to spell, and I have my own month once a year. People often ask if I was born in June; and when I respond, "No, I'm a December baby," they laugh. My mother was born in June, so perhaps that was her motivation in choosing my name.

In biblical times, a name was often an indication of a person's character, nature and ability. People went by their first name and were identified as Shammua son of Zaccur; Shaphat son of Hori; Caleb son of Jephunneh; and so on. Their names had profound meaning, such as Joshua, whose name meant "the Lord saves"; and Hoshea, which means "salvation." In the book of Ruth, she decided her name should be Mara (because her life had become bitter).

Many Christian parents name their children after positive role models from the Bible. Their hope is that it will influence their child's life as they grow and take their place in society. Some parents name their baby after a quality they revere and want to grant the child.

When the angel Gabriel gave Mary the news of the impending birth of the child she would bear, she was instructed to name Him Jesus. The Old Testament form was Yeshua or Joshua, which meant "Yahweh is salvation." The name Jesus was a sign that God would save His people (see Matthew 1:21).

When a person's name becomes tainted (think Judas), it carries a stigma that is difficult to erase. As a child of God, I want to keep my name free of blemishes that would reflect badly for the cause of Christ. The name "Christian" means "follower of Christ." My name is June, daughter of the King, and my goal in life is to truly follow Him who saved me.

Whether your name is Shauna, Shawna, Sean or Shaun, the important thing is that you are a son or daughter of the King, Jesus Christ, the name above all names. He came to save you.

Father, thank You for choosing me to be Your own. I want to
live in such a way that all will say, "Look! There goes, _____,
daughter (son) of King Jesus. How she looks like Him!"
May Your love in me make it so.

Journal: Read 1 Corinthians 13:4-6. Although you can't demonstrate these qualities in your own power, you can ask God to manifest them through you, because you are your Father's child. With which love qualities do you most need the Holy Spirit to help you?

_____

_____

_____

_____

_____

_____

_____

_____

YOU CAN CALL ME SAVIOR
by Vicki Heath

Naming a new baby is a really big deal in any family. We spent hours and hours trying to come up with names for our children. We wanted each child to have a special name as well as a family name. Being of Irish descent, we chose "Megan" for our firstborn. Coming up with a middle name was not so hard. From the beginning she was a daddy's girl, so we gave her Lee, my husband's middle name.

When our second child came along, we both easily agreed on Michael Austin. "Michael," after our best friend in seminary, and "Austin," after my father. With two children whose names started with *M*, our third child had to be the same, of course, or he might feel left out. He was born on a Wednesday, so that night at prayer meeting our church family came up with "Mark Robin," "Matthew" and "Bud"; and in the good Baptist way, we voted on their favorite. I am extremely thankful that our number one choice was "Mark," because "Bud" came in a close second!

By the time our fourth child came along, all three siblings had their own opinion as to what he should be called. After much deliberation, we decided to let each of the three give him a name. That is why Mackenzie Charles Thomas has three names. When he started school, it was Mackenzie; but by second grade, he informed his teachers he was now to be called "Charles." This year he seems to have settled on "Mac." I'm glad he had several from which to choose.

Mary, the mother of Jesus, knew exactly what she was going to name her son. "You are to give him the name Jesus." I don't know if He had a favorite. I wonder if He called Himself different names as He was growing up. Manny (Emmanuel) . . . JC? What do you call Jesus? Sometimes I call Him Savior; sometimes He is my Rescuer; sometimes I call Him Friend. Jesus has so many names, it's hard to pick my favorite. Jesus has been all of these things in my life.

Call Him what you want—He will be all you need. Jesus is many different names to all of us, but He is more than just a name; He *is* His name: the Good Shepherd, King of kings, Savior, Redeemer, Prince of Peace. His name brings life and hope. He is the Son of the Lord Most High, named after His father—name above all names . . . Jesus!

Father, help me to daily remember that Your names perfectly
describe who You are, and that You are all I will ever need.

Journal: Describe a time when God, in Christ Jesus, has been your Refuge, your Healer, your All-Sufficient One . . . or any of the other names of God in Scripture.

Group Prayer Requests

first place
4health

Today's Date: _____

Name	Request

Results

_____
_____
_____
_____
_____

our great God

SCRIPTURE MEMORY VERSE
*He will be great and will be called the Son of the Most High.
The Lord God will give him the throne of his father David.*
LUKE 1:32

THE WAY TO BE GREAT

by Carole Lewis

Day
1

Most of us aspire to greatness. We would like to be thought of as "great" in the eyes of our family, neighbors and work associates. The verse above doesn't say that Jesus would be thought of as great, but that He would be great. For you and I to actually be great, we must learn who Jesus really is and what Jesus really does in the lives of those who follow Him.

When I accepted Jesus as my Savior as a 12-year-old girl, the seed of "greatness" was placed inside of me at that time. The Holy Spirit came to make His home in my heart the minute I asked Jesus to come into my life. That seed was there when I married, and it was there as we raised our three children. But because of my strong, stubborn will, the seed remained a seed for many years.

I did not fully surrender to the greatness of the Lord Jesus until I was 42 years old, and I did it at a time when I was bankrupt in every area of my life—spiritually, mentally, emotionally and physically. From the minute I gave Jesus the reins of control in my life that Sunday morning in 1984, He started doing great things in and through me.

Christmas is a perfect time to reflect on greatness and where we are on the scale. We must always remember that there is nothing inside of us that will push us toward greatness but the power of the risen Christ. None of us possesses the qualities of greatness unless we embrace the life of Jesus and do what He does and be who He is.

This is an impossible task without His power working in us. Where would you like to be a year from now? Would you like to be thought of as great to those you love and to those you meet this next year? What can you do to begin?

- Begin spending time each day getting to really know Jesus.
- Study the Bible to learn who Jesus is and what He can and will do in your life.
- Start acting like Jesus in the lives of those you love and meet every day.
- Become a servant.
- Love unconditionally.
- Give sacrificially.

As you and I learn more about Jesus and give up control of our lives to Him, He will make us great and our lives will blossom and bear the fruit of greatness.

Dear Lord, I want Your greatness to be evident in
my life this Christmas season and in the coming year. Help me
learn what a true servant is and how I might be used by You
in the lives of everyone I know.

Journal: What does greatness mean to you? What would your life look like to have your family think of you as great? Your neighbors? Your coworkers? Ask the Lord Jesus to do the necessary work to make His greatness shine through you.

YOUR ROYAL BLOODLINE
by Betha McGee

My dad had a rather dark complexion. He could not understand why people in South Texas would walk up to him and speak Spanish. Dad did not speak Spanish. He was convinced he was of Irish-German descent and spoke German fluently until the beginning of World War II. After Dad's death, my brother did some research into the family history and discovered that Dad had some Portuguese ancestors who had come here from South America before the Mayflower, and were taken along with some Indians as slaves to Africa. There they intermarried with some of the African people and even later with some of the Jewish race. The dark complexion came to Dad honestly—he just didn't know it!

I was excited when I heard! Which one of the tribes of Israel did we come from? My brother had not seen the need to dig for more. I kept thinking how great it would be if we were from the tribe of Judah and we were part of King David's line! I have not yet been able to research things for myself. But wouldn't it be exciting to be in the same lineage as our Lord?

But wait! God tells us that if we are His children, we are "heirs of God and co-heirs with Christ" (Romans 8:16-17). What does it matter what tribe of Israel might have been represented so many hundreds of years ago? I am a child of the King! What could be any better than that! I thank God for my ancestors—but I am more thankful for my relationship with God and His Son—Jesus.

One of these days, I will stand before my Lord, and it will not matter one whit what line I came from. Being with Jesus will make the other things fade away. To think that Mary was told, "He will be great and will be called the Son of the Most High. The Lord God will give him the throne of his father David." We who love the Lord are the winners, regardless of what bloodline shows up on our family tree. Praise the Lord!

Father, I am overwhelmed with gratitude that You adopted me
into Your family. Help me walk worthy of my family name.

Journal: Use a concordance or concordance software to search "God's people" and "spiritual adoption," and see what Scripture says about you. Make some notes about what it means to be in God's family.

THE ONLY GIFT THAT MATTERS
by Carol VanAtta

Every holiday season on Main Street in Gresham, Oregon, the trees are decorated with twinkling lights, giving the street a fairytale feeling, especially at night after all the shops have closed their doors. I look forward to enjoying this peaceful atmosphere each year. The crowds have gone home. Traffic is light. And I always end up with a warm, fuzzy feeling as I enjoy this very special street.

What a difference from the bustling activity of last-minute shoppers hurrying to find those just-right gifts during daylight hours! There's simply no comparison, just as there is no comparison between the peace of Christ and the chaos of our world's increasingly commercialized Christmas. It's so important for us to keep our eyes on the Son of the Most High instead of worrying about high prices and harried people. Unfortunately, one year I failed miserably at keeping Christ in first place. Maybe you've also done that.

My intentions seemed noble at first. I wanted to bless my children with special gifts because we'd been struggling financially, and I'd had to say no to a lot of reasonable requests. But when I took a longer look at the balance in my checkbook, I realized too late that I simply could not purchase the prizes as planned.

Rather than thanking God for what we had, I ended up feeling sorry for myself and angry at the seemingly "happy shoppers" spending money that I didn't have. I'd stepped right into a trap—greed—that's sure to snatch the joy right out of Christmas. I became grumpy. I ate and ate and ate in one useless attempt after another to drown my despair. All I managed to do was make myself and everyone around me more miserable. Instead of being thankful for Christ, I was bitter after every bite.

One evening, I happened to be walking down Main Street. The trees were twinkling. The sky was clear and filled with shimmering stars, and a group of carolers were singing outside a local coffee shop. To my surprise, I'd stumbled into a real-life Christmas card.

As I soaked in the scene, something happened . . . something miraculous. I forgot about me, me, me, and started thinking about Him, Him, Him. As my thoughts turned to the King on His throne, my money dilemma seemed a lot less important. After all, while on earth, Jesus wasn't rich. He didn't have a ton of money or stuff. He was born in a filthy stable and spent His first night in a feed trough, but in the end, He was seated upon the throne of David forever.

As I went home, I determined to change my attitude and in turn my altitude. I was no longer trudging through the holiday season in misery; now I was flying above my problems on the wings of God's grace. I'd rediscovered the key to Christmas—Christ.

I was reminded that we don't need a ton of money or gifts to enjoy Christmas. We've been given the best gift of all—new life through Christ. We don't need to max out our credit cards or purchase extended warranties, because God's love is the one gift that is FREE and will last unbroken forever.

*Father, please help me focus on what really matters. Depending
on Your peace for my contentment, I remain Your grateful child.*

Journal: What do you do to get your eyes on Jesus when you've succumbed to the stresses of the season? Now follow your own advice!

ALL YOU'VE EVER WANTED

by June Chapko

My birthday is four days before Christmas. When I was growing up, I made sure my parents knew what I wanted as a special gift from them. Our family didn't have much money, so I usually received one main gift that covered both birthday and Christmas. One particular year, my heart's desire was a pair of figure skates. We lived by the lake in Michigan, and I could picture myself twirling around in those pretty white skates with pom-poms on the end of the laces. I kept asking and asking, pleading for my desire. I would try to get Dad to commit by saying to him, "Do you promise?" He was wary of making promises he might not be able to keep, so he would respond with, "I will try." My dad rarely broke a promise to me, unless it was out of his control to fulfill it. I knew that if he promised me figure skates, they were as good as mine.

On Christmas morning that year, I couldn't hold off my anticipation for opening the large box bearing my name. I ripped off the snowflake paper and could smell the rich leather of the skates before taking the top off of the box. They were beautiful, right down to the puffy pom-poms on the laces. I hugged my parents, thanking them for their generosity, then quickly raced to don my socks and try on my skates.

I was too young to understand at what cost those skates came to me that Christmas morning. My parents sacrificed something important to grant their daughter her heart's desire and see excitement and happiness on her face as she opened her gift. They gave me a memory that will last forever.

Today's Scripture speaks to my heart in the same way. The angel Gabriel promises Mary that the child she will bear will be great and will be called the Son of the Most High. He promises that the Lord God will give Him the throne! The word "will" is repeated three times. When God makes a promise, we can depend on it coming to pass. Mary trusted that what God said to her would be accomplished (see v. 45). God had promised King David a lasting kingdom (see 2 Samuel 7:16), and that promise was fulfilled in the birth of our Savior Jesus Christ, a direct descendant of David, whose reign will continue throughout eternity. There is no greater gift than that of Jesus Christ. God sacrificed His only Son to bring us eternal happiness in heaven with Him.

Have you unwrapped God's gift of Salvation by receiving Jesus Christ into your heart? If not, you can do that today. It will be a lasting gift into eternity.

Father, I want my heart to desire what You desire;
teach me how to be satisfied with all that You are in Christ
Jesus, and to stop looking elsewhere.

Journal: Write a letter to God, telling Him how wonderful He is. Make it great and glorious; make it heartfelt and emotion-filled, because He deserves your highest praise.

THE ULTIMATE MENTOR
by Paulette McDonald

There are days when I feel as though I need to have more purpose in my life and some days when I don't feel as though I have any purpose, even as a believer. But, when you study the life of Jesus, your feelings begin to change. Jesus was great in many ways. He was the ultimate mentor.

Jesus taught with parables—spiritual lessons through earthly word pictures. Just think of what a purpose we have in being taught about Jesus. By doing our Bible studies, our eyes are opened and our hearts are softened to the circumstances around us. Once we learn more about Jesus, we have a bigger purpose in teaching others about our Lord, the Son of the Most High.

Jesus also revealed the power of God in the lives of others. This really hit me one day. Wow, this is so important! The Christmas season may be one of the few opportunities we have during the year to introduce ourselves to people and let them know that Jesus loves them. The biggest revelation is not only that Jesus loves them, but that we are willing to invest our lives and our time into the lives of others. As a result, they may join our Bible study group, join our church, get baptized, and possibly reveal the power of God to someone else.

Jesus was and still is the only perfect example we have to live our life. It is so powerful to hear testimonials of others and the mighty works that Jesus has done in their lives. The Holy Spirit shows up in these testimonials and tugs on the hearts of those struggling with the same strongholds. It was during one such powerful testimony that the Holy Spirit spoke to me, "It's not about purpose; it's about opportunity."

Every day we have the opportunity to focus on the same awesome opportunity Jesus gave us to be mentors. The best part about it is that we do not have to look for these people; the Son of the Most High will send them to us.

Father, I'm so grateful for the opportunities You give
me to tell others about You. Help me look for ways to
pass on what I know about You so that others can have new
life through You. In Jesus' name.

Journal: What's the next right thing you can do to make the most of the opportunities God gives you? List names of people who need to hear about Jesus from you and neglected "tools" in your First Place 4 Health arsenal you need to pick up and start using again.

Day
6

ALL I WANT FOR CHRISTMAS
by Vicki Heath

It's been a long time since someone asked me what I wanted for Christmas. It's been a long time since I made a Christmas list like when I was a little girl. I have decided this year I am going to change that; I'm making a list and submitting it to my heavenly Father who is in the business of giving. He gave His throne to Jesus, and Jesus is there at the right hand of the Father, telling our heavenly Father just what we need. He is the giver of every good and perfect gift (see James 1:17).

The main thing I want: an MHVR player—a Mind and Heart Video Recorder to permanently record impressions on my mind and heart. If I could just capture Christmas moments in my mind and heart forever! If I could just keep my children small! If I could always have focused thoughts on Jesus, God's perfect gift! If I could record the smiles, laughter, lights and stars . . . permanently!

I am asking God to give me a heart to remember others and to remember the *best* things about my family, not focus on the dysfunctional things. I am asking God for an *abundance* of grace, love and mercy. I am asking God to renew my mind by the power of the Holy Spirit that I may have a new way of thinking this year and that it might be permanent! I believe God wants to bless His children at Christmas, so I'm asking!

"If you, then, though you are evil, know how to give good gifts to your children, how much more will your Father in heaven give good gifts to those who ask him!" (Matthew 7:11). How about you? What do you want for Christmas? He is on His throne just waiting to hear.

*Father God, please give me a heart that loves others with
Your love. And while You're at it, please give me an abundance
of Your grace and mercy. And please make it permanent!*

Journal: When it comes to your heavenly Father, you're never too old to make a Christmas wish list. Just remember to ask Him to tell You what's on His heart and write it down. The Holy Spirit will take it from there!

DIE BEFORE YOU DIE
by Vicki Heath

While Jesus accomplished great things during His ministry and short 33 years here on earth, His greatest accomplishment did not occur until He surrendered to His death. In order for us to live, He had to die. He was not recognized for who He really was until after the crucifixion. He did not ascend to the promised "throne of his father David" until after His life here on earth was over. He is now called the "Son of the Most High" but He was not then. He was scorned and rejected, spat upon and despised. They did not recognize who He was.

And so may it be with us. Some of us may accomplish great things for the Kingdom while here on this earth, but the greatest accomplishment for the Lord will only come one way—by the way of the cross. The apostle Paul says it this way in Galatians 2:20: "I have been crucified with Christ and I no longer live, but Christ lives in me. The life I live in the body, I live by faith in the Son of God, who loved me and gave himself for me."

As I die to self every day, Christ will accomplish great things through me. As I lay aside my ego and appetite, He will live through me. For me personally, I have to intentionally set aside my body daily for crucifixion. I usually do this during my quiet time every morning with the Lord. If not, my old self will rise up and my ego will rule me and my day. My ego says things like, "Live for yourself today—you deserve it!" Not true! We deserve death and hell! Dying to self must be a lifelong decision we practice daily.

Jesus said, "Whoever loses his life for me will find it" (Matthew 16:25). If you have not come to the point of total surrender to Christ, do it today. My son, Michael, says it this way: die before you die. Die to self and let Him be recognized as great. Give Him the place of honor in your life: the throne of your heart.

Father, help me die to myself today and live for You; I can't do
this on my own, so I ask You to show Yourself great in me.

Journal: What ego appetites, in every area of your life, do you need to surrender to your great God? Ask God to resurrect your appetite for Him, His will and His Word.

Group Prayer Requests

first place
4health

Today's Date: _____

Name	Request

Results

_____
_____
_____
_____
_____

a new
direction

SCRIPTURE MEMORY VERSE
He put a new song in my mouth, a hymn of praise to our God
PSALM 40:3

CHRISTMAS GIFTS

Day
1

by Carole Lewis

The Christmas of 2008 found us facing the new year with our home on Galveston Bay destroyed by Hurricane Ike. We had it torn down during the month of December, and our Christmas cards that year showed Johnny and me standing on the muddy bulldozer with the caption, "A New Chapter Begins." That was probably the most dramatic new year we have ever experienced, but as I look back, I am reminded of the truth of Psalm 40:3. God has truly put a new song in my mouth and a hymn of praise to His faithfulness in our lives.

God provided, for the year 2009, a beautiful townhome of a friend that was fully furnished. In December of that year, He provided a way for us to purchase a townhome in the same subdivision. Our son, John, was available to serve as the contractor to oversee the remodeling, which was such a blessing. God provided two great sub-contractors, Max and Jorge, to do all the excellent work on our new home.

My greatest concern and prayer was for my friend Linda to sell her townhome quickly after we moved. We moved out on April 1, and Linda closed on the sale of her townhome on May 17, just six weeks after we moved! And this is during a time when approximately 15 townhomes are for sale in our subdivision.

God had a new direction for our life, and He used the calamity of Hurricane Ike to nudge us in the direction and new plan He had for us. I am convinced that we would never have left the bay unless our home was totally destroyed.

It has been such a blessing to be closer to Johnny as he has gone through five months of chemo. It would have been totally impossible to run home the 46 miles to the bay when he needed me. We have been blessed to live 10 minutes away from our kids and from my office. We are completely at peace and in love with our new home.

My takeaway is that James 1 is completely true. If we "Count it all joy when we face various trials," our God will use those trials to "put a new song in our mouth."

Dear Lord, help us when we face trials of many kinds
to trust You to bring us out on the other side. Thank You for
putting a new song in our mouth when we emerge
victorious over the trials we all face.

Journal: Write in your journal about the worst trial you have gone through and how God carried you through to the other side and put a new song in your mouth. Write a hymn of praise to Him.

A NEW BOSS
by Bev Schwind

I glanced up from reading my book as the man carrying a brown lunch bag sat down across from me. The seating arrangement was more like an airport than a physician's office. Seven other men were sitting in the waiting room of the Veteran's hospital. My husband was having his hearing checked.

The man sitting almost knee to knee with me wore a faded baseball cap that said, "Friend of Jesus." His western boots showed much use.

"Did you bring a lunch?" I asked.

"No, ma'am, it is my hearing aid; it needs workin' on."

"I like your cap," I said to extend the conversation.

"Yes, ma'am," he said with a smile. "He became my friend 45 years ago." His eyes danced like it had happened yesterday.

"I played the guitar and fiddle in a band, and we had a New Year's Eve booking. I got off work early, because it was beginning to snow hard and it was a holiday coming on. I stopped at the bar as usual and had a few beers with the guys.

"My wife liked going to church and that is where she planned to go on New Year's Eve. Her cousins were going to pick her up, as I told her more than once I did not want anything to do with her God. I could not see Him, but I could see my beer. Outside, the weather was getting worse, and a phone call told me that our band engagement had been cancelled.

"My cousin called and said he couldn't get his car out and wanted to know if I could drive them to church, and if I stayed and played music, he would give me the $50 I had planned on. 'Fifty dollars is fifty dollars,' I said, and I consented to drive."

By this time the other men in the waiting room were involved with the story. I watched them leaning in to hear when my new friend lowered his voice to tell me something.

He laughed as he told me how he played the music but did not want the preacher to come near him. "That man preached and something happened to me; I wasn't thinking about beer anymore, but about Jesus. I ended up surrendering my life to Him on New Year's Eve. I used to sing in bars and now I sing for a different owner."

He handed me his business card that was for a group of four who were serving the Lord through a music ministry. They were all members of his family.

"You certainly started out the New Year right," I commented.

My husband walked out as the story ended. I introduced him to the man.

"I see you know my friend," my husband said as he looked at the man's cap and shook his hand.

I came away refreshed by the testimony of praise from the unknown man in the waiting room.

Lord, I want to be like the man who wears a "Friend of Jesus" cap. Help me to be as open and eager as he is to talk about You to strangers. I'm excited to see who You will bring my way so that I can tell them the reason for the hope within me.

Journal: Write about the last time you talked to someone about Jesus, and what transpired. If it's been awhile, make your next conversation—with a family member, a coworker or a stranger—about the One who has made all the difference in your life.

SING A NEW SONG
by Charlotte Davis

I was the fifth of six children, and my family didn't have a lot of material things when I was growing up, but music filled our home. My father was a radio disc jockey who answered God's call to preach His Word when he was in his mid-twenties. Though his job as a DJ in a small Louisiana town didn't pay well (and his bi-vocational pastor position at a tiny country church paid much less), he did have the terrific benefit of getting free "used" records (yes, those vinyl discs) at his job. In the 1960s, radio stations didn't specialize in certain genres of music like they do now, so he had everything from Tom Jones to The Association to Bob Wills to The Blackwood Brothers!

When I was two years old, we moved to Arkansas, where Daddy took his first full-time pastorate. All of those records came with us. I grew up playing them over and over, singing at the top of my lungs. Over the years, my dad got children's and youth choirs going in our small church, and I was the first one to show up for practice. He also loved to sing at church, and he had a fantastic baritone voice. Talk about a package deal—a pastor who could sing! Everyone said he sounded like Jim Reeves!

Daddy always encouraged his kids to sing, too, and play the piano and play in the school band. However, he always emphasized the importance of using musical talents, abilities and tools to serve God—those gifts came *from* Him and should be used *for* Him. When other pastors of that day were resisting the use of "canned music" in worship services, Daddy was giddily running the reel-to-reel background tape for our children's choir's Fourth of July musical!

In 1995, my dad began experiencing heart problems that required heart by-pass surgery. The doctors told him to lose weight to improve his health. That same year, I began my first First Place 4 Health group, and he joined it. He lost more than 20 pounds and was a great supporter of the program, not to mention a great advertisement!

My precious daddy went home to be with the Lord earlier this year, at the age of 81. At the funeral, we played a CD of him singing, along with the traditional slide show of pictures to honor his life. Sweet notes and words from songs like "He Touched Me" and "Prayer Is the Key to Heaven" filled the church. Daddy was singing in *two* places that day!

The Sunday after the funeral, I resumed my spot on the worship team at our church and sang a "new song" with everything I had in me. Though this was a new chapter in my life, and I wasn't sure how things were going to be, with this gaping hole left by my father's death, I knew God had a plan and was still in control. Tears came, but I wanted to praise the Lord in the best way I could, because He deserves it, and Daddy would certainly expect it!

Father, music is one of Your great gifts. Thank You for
how music brings us into Your throne room and helps our hearts
worship You in Spirit and in truth.

Journal: Ask the Holy Spirit to give you a "new song" to sing or pray to the Lord. The first step is to desire God above all else and spend time with Him: "You will seek me and find me when you seek me with all your heart" (Jeremiah 29:13).

ALL THINGS NEW
by Jenn Krogh

"New." The word brings images of all kinds of exciting things, doesn't it? New job, new car, new friend, new clothes, New Year, new beginnings!

Back in January 2002, I began a new journey. I became a leader of First Place 4 Health in my church. It was a new program, and no one was familiar with it where I live. In October of that same year, I made the commitment to be the First Place 4 Health Networking Leader for Wisconsin. It was an exciting time, and a bit scary stepping into all that newness. I began new relationships as I met other leaders in various cities. It was a new experience planning meetings and events held in various churches around the state. I belong to a small church, so I gained a new understanding of how larger churches operate as I worked with leaders from those congregations.

All of this brought a new song in my mouth! A new adventure had begun, and it has continued all these years. Every step is new, and God has an amazing way of breathing freshness into each one of those steps. Every 12 weeks is a new session, bringing new faces. But even more than that, God is working in and through my heart each day, bringing into it new life. My eyes see new things and my mind is being made new by the power of His Word. My heart is being renewed daily by the power of His Holy Spirit.

A synonym for "new" describes things that have not existed or have not been known or seen before. God is so exciting! He breathes new life into those seeking Him. I have witnessed the "new" physical bodies of members who have embraced the Live It plan and made it their lifestyle. I have watched God break the chains of emotional bondage in individuals who have learned to trust Him, and then seen a new sparkle in their eyes and a smile to match. I have seen First Place 4 Health members experience renewal in their marriages that were on the verge of collapse, and receive a freshness in their relationships that were stagnant without the power of the risen Lord.

As we begin this New Year, my personal desire is to begin each day with the same enthusiasm as the New Year celebration. I want to experience our Lord in every choice and decision I make. My mouth has a new song of praise every time I put my trust in Him. My heart has a new song as I witness others "see and fear and put their trust in Him."

Father, this new year, help me daily die to my petty
desires that can never satisfy. I want to be able to truly say, along
with the psalmist, "As the deer pants for streams of water, so my
soul pants for you, O God" (Psalm 42:1)

Journal: What is most problematic for you? Negative self-talk, emotional overreaction to stress, unwise food choices, neglect of your relationship with God? Give your struggle to God and ask the Holy Spirit for a new beginning.

A MELODY DIVINE
by Karrie Smyth

Day 5

I love new beginnings! New mercies every morning. New to-do lists each week. New years full of potential and renewed commitment. New works of Christ in me. As I look back over the years and what Christ has been accomplishing in me, I learn new songs of praise to sing to Him. Romans 12:1 tells me that when I place my life before God as an offering, that is my spiritual act of worship. When I look back and observe the ways that God has been moving in my life, I begin to see what song He has been singing over me and add my voice to the melody. Let's see if I can show you what I mean.

One of the songs the Lord has put in my mouth comes from Psalm 113:9: "He settles the barren woman in her home as a happy mother of children. Praise the LORD." Over the years, He has added new layers of harmonies. First, He gave me my son. Then, He gave me my daughter. Later, He gave me happiness; and now, I see Him settling me in my home. I sing this song of praise to our God!

Sometimes the song of praise has had a minor sound to it. Though I had been a Christian for many years, God took me through a season where He stripped me bare of everything that I was holding on to—except Him. Through those years, He taught me to sing, "The LORD is my rock, my fortress and my deliverer; my God is my rock, in whom I take refuge. He is my shield and the horn of my salvation, my stronghold" (Psalm 18:2). When He brought me out of this season, He added the chorus, "He reached down from on high and took hold of me; he drew me out of deep waters. . . . He brought me out into a spacious place; he rescued me because he delighted in me" (Psalm 18:16,19).

As I begin to recognize this anthem, I hear some recurring strains: "Let us not become weary in doing good, for at the proper time we will reap a harvest if we do not give up" (Galatians 6:9), and "I am the LORD, your God, who takes hold of your right hand and says to you, Do not fear; I will help you" (Isaiah 41:13).

Whether you're singing from the top of the mountain or you're journeying through a dark valley, you can bet that God has a song of praise to put in your mouth. The contrast between high notes and low gives wonderful richness to the song. Sing it back to Him. Sing it to those around you. Many will see and fear the Lord and put their trust in God as your life sings a song of praise.

Father, what new thing do You want to do in me today? My hope is in You alone. I'm looking forward to singing the songs You put in my mouth this new year, and I will sing them back to You with a grateful heart.

Journal: What recurring "melody" is God showing you? Maybe you just heard it today. Write about the song of praise and sing or pray it back to God.

GOD OF THE DO-OVER

by Kathlee Coleman

On December 27, 2005, I was looking back at a year of struggle to ful-fill my resolution to the Lord to keep up a regular quiet time. I had also not kept my resolution to lose excess weight by eating healthier and ex-ercising. Feeling miserable, I felt like giving up. I had been a member and leader of a First Place 4 Health group for two years and was not a good example to my group of someone who followed through on her commitment. I decided to stop trying and attempt to be happy at a weight of over 200 pounds.

The next day I was praying during my quiet time (I had renewed my commitment to that!). God put it on my heart that I needed to give Him another chance. He convicted me that I had not given any of my weight-loss efforts 100 percent. The Lord gently redirected my heart from my self-centered misery to focusing on developing a healthy tem-ple of the Holy Spirit. I was still a bit rebellious toward the idea and told the Lord that He had this one last chance. Silly me!

I realized that New Year's resolutions were not what I needed. I needed a change in the "song" that my heart sings. I needed to stop singing the old "songs" that said I would never succeed. Those songs said that whenever life got difficult, I'd run back to my old habits. The new "song" the Lord gave me was one of success through His help. The new song says that even when difficulties come, you can rely on God to give you the strength to overcome. You do not have to return to your old ways of handling stress (eating!). You can run to the Lord to sustain you in those times.

That day I began to research additional accountability through on-line friendships. That, in addition to my local First Place 4 Health group, helped me start the lifestyle of consistency. I stopped looking at my efforts as dieting and started looking at them as healthy lifestyle changes that would lead to a life lived in a way that was good, pleasing and acceptable to the Lord.

Walking along this road has not always been easy. I've even gained back some weight that I lost. But the truths I've learned have not left me. Nor has God's work in me been for me alone. The Lord has used my testimony to help others have hope and trust in the Lord. I am grateful and humbled that He chose to work in me in such a way.

Father, even when I give up on myself, You never
give up on me. Thank You for being the God of the do-over
(and over and over). I get it now! Only when You lead me will I
ever walk in that good, pleasing and acceptable way.
So here I am again, asking You to do what You do best.
Thank You for Your new mercies every day.

Journal: Write about God's mercies to you today as you walk with Him. Or maybe you need to ask Him to lead you back to the pathway from which you've strayed. He will be more than happy to help you start anew.

NEW YEAR'S RESOLUTION
by Martha Rogers

Day
7

For many years, I made resolutions for the New Year. After several weeks, most of those resolutions were broken and dropped by the wayside. After being in First Place 4 Health several years and learning about long-term and short-term goals, I dropped the resolutions.

Now I set goals for myself at the beginning of the year. The short-term goals are those I want to accomplish within a few months, while the long-term goals will take the year or maybe longer to accomplish. I claimed Galatians 6:9, "Let us not become weary in doing good, for at the proper time we will reap a harvest if we do not give up," as my life verse, to keep me on track so I wouldn't give up.

The verse for this week has put a new perspective on those goals. The Lord puts a new song in my mouth every morning to praise Him and thank Him for all He has done and for what He has planned for that day. Each day is a new gift from Him to work toward my goals as I put my trust in Him.

When others see the song in our hearts and hear the song from our lips, they will be drawn closer to Him. We make it our goal to please the Lord in whatever we do, wherever we are, and with whomever we meet. Let us sing that new song with joy in our hearts. May our voices be lifted in a praise song to our Lord every day.

One of the great things about First Place 4 Health is the Bible study. Spending time with the Lord in prayer and reading the Scriptures are also a part of the plan to give us a well-balanced lifestyle. When we walk with the Lord daily in the light of His Word, we find the day goes easier, and it becomes a habit to trust and obey.

A day begun with prayer and praise as we study the Scripture and read His Word will not come unraveled and fall apart. As you begin this year, what is the song He has put in your mouth? What do you want to accomplish this year? With the "Give God a Year" plan, not only can you work toward the goals you set, but you can also depend on the Lord to accomplish His will in your life.

Father, I love to sing the songs You put in my mouth.
Your words bring light and life to my soul. Help me hear what
You are telling me today, and thank You for the beginning of a
new year, a new day, to praise Your name.

Journal: What are your long-term goals for a healthier life? What are your short-term goals to help keep you focused on getting there? Ask God to show you the next step toward your goal.

Group Prayer Requests

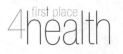

Today's Date: _____

Name	Request

Results

_____

_____

_____

_____

_____

the light of the world

SCRIPTURE MEMORY VERSE

Yet I am writing you a new command; its truth is seen in him and you, because the darkness is passing and the true light is already shining.

1 JOHN 2:8

WHEN THE LIGHT IS BRIGHTEST
by Carole Lewis

Day
1

I am so grateful that I have lived long enough to experience the truth of this verse as Johnny and I have faced dark times. We went through bankruptcy in 1984, Johnny was diagnosed with stage 4 prostate cancer in 1997, our daughter Shari was killed by a drunk driver in 2001, and our home was destroyed by Hurricane Ike in 2008. Add to that the regular difficulties of life, like caring for my mom the last three years of her life while driving 100 miles each day to work and back home, not to mention the ongoing "battle of the bulge" all of us in First Place 4 Health face.

I have learned that in this life we will always be dealing with something difficult. I have also learned that those are the times when God will shine most brightly in our lives . . . *if we will let Him.* Psalm 139:11-12 says it best: "If I say, 'Surely the darkness will hide me and the light become night around me,' even the darkness will not be dark to you; the night will shine like the day, for darkness is as light to you."

As Christians, we would hope that when we go through dark times, we will be able to shine brightly, reflecting God's light to our lost world. The light of Christ shining in our lives during our dark times can serve as a reminder to others that God can be trusted when they, too, walk through a dark time.

God has used every bad and painful experience that we have ever walked through to show Himself faithful to us. Johnny and I are truly thankful that we have been given the opportunity to experience the love and faithfulness of God as we have walked this cancer journey. Our marriage is sweeter and more precious than it ever was before this awful disease. We don't waste a minute being angry, and we are grateful for every minute we have together. We celebrated 50 years of marriage in 2009, when we never dreamed that would be a possibility after his diagnosis in 1997.

God shines the brightest when we walk through the dark times. I truly believe that God doesn't take it lightly when His children suffer. Even though we live in a fallen world, God is able to redeem our lives from the pit in which we may find ourselves: "Praise the Lord, O my soul . . . who redeems your life from the pit and crowns you with love and compassion" (Psalm 103:2,4). He sets our feet on a rock and gives us a firm place to stand: "He lifted me out of the slimy pit, out of the mud and mire; he set my feet on a rock and gave me a firm place to stand" (Psalm 40:2).

Dear Lord, help me to see the dark
times of my life as a means for Your light to shine
through me to lead others to trust in You. Thank You
for being there with me every time I go through
a dark period. Thank You for always bringing
Your light into my darkness and for bringing
me out on the other side.

Journal: Write about some of the dark periods of your own life and reflect on how Jesus brought light to your situation. Thank Him for His faithfulness.

LIGHT WALKING
by Bev Schwind

This was the third year we were doing the First Place 4 Health program at the church. Each class was filled with different expectations. Some of the people did not believe in their hearts they could reach their goals, but through the program they began to believe in their self-worth and that God would help them.

Becky, a young mother with a six-month-old baby boy, wanted to attend the meetings but didn't have a baby-sitter, as her husband worked during that time. We welcomed them both into the group. We went around the table, with the 10 women introducing themselves and telling their goals. Becky shared openly with us that she was bulimic and purged on a regular basis. She wanted the help and support of the group while learning to eat nutritious foods.

As a leader, I had not dealt with bulimic situations, but God provided. An older lady looked at Becky and said, "I used to purge too." Becky looked at her and immediately shot a question back to her. "Are you over it?" The woman told her story that she had started this terrible addiction when a group of high school girls thought it fun years ago. She joined them, but did not realize they had not continued on with the habit. But she did, and when she married, she did this in secret.

By chance, she found an article about bulimia, realized it had a name and that she was headed for trouble unless she could stop. There was not much information and she had no one she felt she could tell. Through her relationship with the Lord, and the article she had found, she began to win over the addiction. "I still fight the urge at times," she confessed, "but I am able to dismiss the temptation through prayer." Becky was relieved to see and talk with a person who had recovered from bulimia and wanted to lose weight.

Through the year, Becky grew stronger and victorious. The class was encouraging to one another and showed great love. The next year, Becky told me she would not be in class, as she was going back to college, having dropped out before because of her addiction.

I did not see Becky for several years, and then one day she was in my life again. This time she looked beautiful and had two sons—a two-year-old and a four-year-old. Her husband was so proud of his boys and Becky. Through the love of Christ and supportive people, the darkness in Becky's life had disappeared and her new life in Christ was shining for all to see. The new year would also see Becky graduating from college.

Becky and her family have moved away, but I still hear from her on occasion. One day, I got an exciting phone call from Becky, who told me to watch the *700 Club* on television and see her story. She had believed and received a victory!

Lord, thank You for shining Your light in the dark places of my life. I want to shine more and more for You this year. Help me live in such a way that I never quench Your light in me.

Journal: Write about your latest miracle from God—it could be a new way of seeing; a new way of being; a new way of living—all because He gives you the victory. Dedicate this new year to walking in His marvelous light.

IS THE LIGHT ON?
by June Chapko

My Bible is my life workbook, evidenced by highlighted passages, underscoring, exclamation marks and hastily sketched light bulbs indicating those "aha!" moments when God turns the light of His Word on in my life. I can open my Bible to most any Old Testament or New Testament book and locate favorite verses, salvation passages and well-worn verses in the psalms that I've visited on many occasions. I linger over my personal notes to work on a discipline pointed out to me by the Holy Spirit. They beckon my heart during my quiet moments with God, and I realize as the New Year begins that I have added yet another life workbook to my spiritual growth library.

I discovered some years ago that replacing my Bible every five or six years is something I must do in order to continue growing spiritually. When I search the well-marked passages and sections, I begin to presume I know a truth so well that I am unable to grasp anything new in it. The "aha!" sketches become less frequent, and my ability to take ownership of the new command God has just for me becomes more difficult.

This is the fifth year in my current Bible, and as is my tradition on New Year's Eve, I go through it and savor the truth He has shown me through the beautiful examples of God's character, mercy and love. From the creation in Genesis (see Genesis 1–2) through the promise that God will wipe away every tear, and death shall be no more (see Revelation 21:4), I realize that the darkness is passing and my Lord Jesus, the true Light, is already shining. I look for the "light bulbs" that remind me to walk in the new thing He reveals. I find many of my First Place 4 Health memory verses highlighted and close my eyes to recall them silently. I feast on the fruit of the Spirit, examining myself for evidence of His presence in my life. Love is both the old and new commandment He wants to see in me.

I'm hungry for His Word. I pick up the new Bible I bought myself for Christmas and quietly ask God to bless my time spent in reading and studying His Word in this as-yet-unmarked Bible. I encourage the Holy Spirit to give me understanding each time I take my place for my appointment with the Lord. I invite Jesus to shine His light on the truth I need to learn in the years ahead. My markers lie still, a pen rests on the table by my chair. When I begin my journey through this Bible, I will see familiar verses and truths, but God will show them to me in a new perspective, free from old notes and ideas.

Do you sense the darkness passing as the old year fades away and a new one begins? Get ready, because the true light is already shining.

Father, I am hungry for more of the light of Your
Word in this new year. Give me understanding as I read and
meditate on what You say. I ask You, Holy Spirit, to
examine the health of my heart so that it can become more
Light-filled and conformed to Your Son.

Journal: By now you're in the habit of creating a "life workbook" through your journal entries. If you're still hit and miss with it, start writing again today. It's a great way to actually see God's presence, and you never have to change a light bulb!

_____

_____

_____

_____

_____

_____

_____

SHINE YOUR LIGHT, LORD!
by June Chapko

Having been in First Place 4 Health since the mid 1990s as a leader, I learned/taught the basics of the program in the old format when it was simply called First Place. I studied the Live It, made good strides in fulfilling the nine commitments, utilized the Fact Sheet to record my meals and followed the plan pretty well. I grew comfortable in thinking I was successful as I lost weight, even though I still had not reached my goal weight.

Over the years, as First Place 4 Health changed by updating the program as more health knowledge became available, I adapted to those changes, albeit a little hesitantly. Change can be disconcerting to some; and while it seems awkward at times, we all know that sometimes change is necessary and good. The basics of First Place 4 Health still contain the same principles as in the beginning. While we don't check off our nine commitments now, they are built into the four areas of mental, physical, spiritual and emotional living. The Fact Sheet was revised and given the appropriate name of Live It Tracker. The Live It Food Plan was updated to include a plan for everyone, not just those dealing with diabetes. First Place 4 Health was and is a good, sound Christian health program for those who desire a lasting way to balanced living.

I look now at the new First Place 4 Health program and realize that here God has provided me a new way to follow the old plan. It was and is built upon the truth of His Word. The promises He gave, the verses I have memorized, the work He began in me, and the disciplines I have learned are still valid. He didn't do away with the old; He transformed it into the new. When I do my Bible study each morning, and as I review my memory verses each day during my meditation and prayer time throughout the week, in all of these I see God's truth. Now, He wants to see it in *me*! He wants His light to shine out so that others will take notice and ask what I've been doing to lose weight. That will be the testimony that will change people's hearts and minds about Christ Jesus. When we become a beacon that reflects Jesus Christ; as we progressively live the Word by walking in obedience to the principles God has provided; others will see our progress and want to be a part of what we're doing. I desire to lead others out of darkness and into the light. The way to do that is to continue following the plan, depending on Christ for my strength, and allowing His light to shine through me.

Is God's truth seen in you? Walk in what you know and ask Him to provide strength to learn the rest.

*Jesus, shine Your light through me so that others who
are walking in darkness will run to You. May Your kingdom
come, may Your will be done in earth as it is in heaven.*

Journal: Write about how you are learning to rely on God's strength more and more to make good health choices. How do you see mind, body, emotions and spirit linked in this regard?

LIFE IN GOD'S HANDS
by Lisa Lewis

Day
5

There are times, when I am in the darkness, that instead of trusting God and looking to the true Light, I struggle and fight to fix it in my own power. Even when I know it is out of my hands.

When our oldest child was about four, we decided we wanted to have another baby. It didn't take long before I was pregnant. I was so excited! At about six weeks, I started having severe pain on my right side. After several days of the pain getting worse and worse, plus other symptoms, I went to the doctor and found out the pregnancy was ectopic. I lost that child and was heartbroken.

It wasn't long before I was pregnant again and everything seemed fine. Then at about six weeks, I miscarried. I started to lose hope that we would be able to have any more children. Surgeries during these two pregnancies reduced my chance of getting pregnant by 50 percent. However, 50 percent is plenty for God, and I got pregnant again. I was considered high risk at this point, so I went to the doctor at six weeks. They used a device that would enable us to hear the baby's heartbeat; but after trying for about five minutes, we were not able to hear anything. The nurse left and got the doctor. He came in and searched for a heartbeat, with no success. He told me that based on the level of HCG (pregnancy hormone) indicated in my blood tests, we should be able to hear the heartbeat by now. It was late on Friday afternoon, so he recommended I go home and come back on Monday, and we would try again and also do an ultrasound.

I don't know how I answered him or paid my bill or made my way to my car. Alone, I sat in my car sobbing. How was I going to sit at home all weekend thinking my baby had died? After about 10 minutes of just sitting there and crying, I said to myself, *Well, how dumb is this? Lisa, what are you doing? This is too big for you. Why don't you trust God with this? Give it to Him and let it go.* So I started praying. As I prayed, the peace that came over me is indescribable. I drove home and made it through the weekend fine.

When I went back to the doctor on Monday, I saw my beautiful little boy's heart beating on the sonogram, my little boy who is now 6' 1" and 195 pounds. My hope meter was at an all-time low for a little while; but when I trusted God, He filled it back up and then blessed me in a big way with a healthy child.

If we trust God in our darkness, His true light will shine in our life.

Lord, help me to trust You in all circumstances, to let go
and let You have control of my life and to believe that You have a
plan and a hope for my future (see Jeremiah 29:11).

Journal: What are you holding on to and struggling with when what you need to do is let go and let God? Thank Him for His sovereignty in your life, and for His peace that passes all human understanding.

LEAVING THE DARKNESS OF SELF-WILL
by Luanne Blackburn

I went to a graduation ceremony recently that was unlike any I had been to before. It was for a technical college that offers two-year programs in health-related fields. A relative of mine was receiving her practical nursing degree. Most of the 70 graduates appeared to be 20-somethings, many of them single parents, with a sprinkling of middle-aged people seeking a late career change.

Christina, one of the student speakers, told the incredible story of how she got to this day. Just a few years before, she was huddled in a dark apartment in Texas, riding out a hurricane. Scared and alone, she cradled her baby girl, born just two weeks prior. Her boyfriend, the father of her baby, had beaten her again. "I was lost in the darkness of my own personal hurricane," she said. Utterly defeated, she made a desperate call to her mother in Indiana.

Having children the same age as Christina, I imagined the backstory to this phone call: rebellious teenager; concerned parents; unheeded warnings; estrangement; an out-of-wedlock pregnancy. When Christina picked up that phone and finally got through, her mom had no rebuke. She simply said, "Come home." Two days later, the mother arrived in Texas, packed up her daughter and granddaughter, and gave Christina a second chance at life. Beaming proudly from the podium, Christina fully acknowledged that she was only there because of the grace and forgiveness shown to her on a dark Texas day.

Aren't we all like this young lady, at times lost in the darkness of hurricanes of our own making? We know God loves us and wants what is best for us. We know that Christ died for us. Yet we insist on doing things our own way. His Word shines a light on the right path for our lives, but so often we choose the dark path of our own will. We come to our First Place 4 Health meetings, but we don't follow the Live It plan.

We enjoy the Bible study and fellowship with other members, but we don't pick up the phone to encourage someone we know is having a difficult time. We step on the scale week after week, hoping we have lost weight, yet we won't fill out a Live It Tracker or exercise our bodies.

What kept Christina from calling her mother before her situation became so desperate? Maybe she couldn't admit she was wrong. Perhaps she was afraid of hearing, "I told you so." But I'll bet her mom had been waiting for that call for years, hoping that Christina was finally ready to come home, to receive the forgiveness she was so willing to give. Our God is a God of second chances. One of my big takeaways from a recent First Place 4 Health session was that Christ will never chide us or scold us when we come to Him in our weakness. He is always waiting for us to turn our backs on sin and come home.

With Christ, every day is New Year's Day. We can always make a fresh start. We can leave behind the darkness of our disobedience and run to Him into the true light of His love.

Father, so often I choose the dark path of my own will.
I want a fresh start. So I am running toward the light of Your
love. To stay there will require some new choices. So I
ask You to take control once again and lead me back to health
in mind, body, emotions and spirit.

Journal: Is there something in your First Place 4 Health plan that needs a fresh start? Write about it and surrender it to the Lord.

RENOVATED BY GOD
by Paulette McDonald

Day
7

Have you ever painted a dark-colored room to a fresh, light color? I have done a lot of painting while renovating several houses. One day as I painted, I began to pray. Then the Holy Spirit began to reveal that the Lord wants to show us how to prepare and paint the room that is our body— what colors to put in our room, how to prepare to paint and how many coats of paint our room needs, as well as what we will need for our room.

Sometimes before you paint a room in a house, there are holes to patch first. The needed patches in us may be emotional, mental, physical or spiritual in nature. Perhaps in the first few months of following a new way of living, you will see healing take place but not necessarily a huge weight loss. The Lord is just patching and caulking the room that is your body.

In my house renovations, I've noticed that, sometimes, older rooms have cracked walls that need a little wood filler. Our body may sustain cracks of discouragement that get filled by encouraging one another and praying for one another. Or rather than cracks to be filled, we wear a pattern of wallpaper that needs to be removed. We might have to tear down some of our layers of darkness before the painting process so that we will be open to the truth of God's Word and a life full of light.

Before you begin to paint inside a house, you have to have the right equipment to create the desired texture. The Bible is the right equipment God wants us to use to get the desired texture in us. You can lose weight, gain it back and stay on a roller coaster of up-and-down weight loss, but if you have God's Word in your heart, there is something that happens to the texture of your walls. Without the Bible, you will continue to search aimlessly for a texture that only Jesus can give you.

Can you guess what color God wants for your room? Think of how beautiful a table full of fruit and vegetables looks. Let's say you are going to paint your room asparagus green. Unfortunately, to get the right color luminosity, the walls need more than one coat. There are going to be times when you will have to give yourself another coat of paint, which is the truth of Scripture. Satan wants us to focus on feelings, and he lies to us through our feelings, but we need to continue to coat our room until the Scriptures become a part of our heart, and the mighty God we serve keeps us from believing the lies.

God wants to be the one to paint our walls. He wants to be a part of the process; but He gives us a choice. We have to choose to want Him and to let the people He has put in our lives help us.

Father, the room of my heart needs some renovation.
Please come in and do whatever will reflect the luminosity
of Jesus. And please help me stay the course in my
ongoing remodel of my physical wellness. Reveal to me the
color and texture that reflects Your beauty.

Journal: Metaphorically speaking, do you need another coat of paint? Do you need to be completely repainted? What color are you going to choose? How will you make sure that God is the one who guides those decisions?

Group Prayer Requests

first place
4health

Today's Date: _____

Name	Request

Results

_____
_____
_____
_____
_____
_____

holiday
survival tips

Maintaining healthy eating habits and an exercise regimen during the holidays can seem like an overwhelming task. Many times, all of our good habits we have worked so hard to develop are thrown out the window as soon as November arrives! Planning ahead for holiday challenges is the key to surviving the holidays with those healthy habits intact. These suggestions will help you experience a healthier holiday season.

FOCUS AND PRIORITIZE

- Take inventory. Identify all the situations (office parties, mall food courts, family gatherings) that make it difficult for you to eat healthy during the holiday season. Make a plan for staying on track in every situation.

- Stay active. Don't mistake being busy for being active. You still need to exercise at least 30 minutes each day. Break it up into smaller sessions throughout the day if you're pressed for time.

- Start a new tradition. Focus on fun activities, not food. Take a walk to see some of the neighborhood decorations, sing some holiday carols, see a play, or volunteer to help those in need.

HEALTHY ACTIVITIES

- Walk more. Maintain a brisk walking pace while you do your holiday shopping. Instead of wasting time looking for a parking spot
  that is closer to the store, take one that is farther away to increase
  your activity (and save you time).

- Join a holiday race. Most cities offer running and walking events
  around the holidays. These events typically not only raise money
  for charity, but they can also help to keep you active on a day that
  would otherwise be filled with overindulgence.

- Volunteer to help a family. Help a mom or dad by offering to take their
  young children for a stroller ride.

- Clean out your closets. Go through any unwanted clothing items in
  your closets and donate the items to a local charity.

PARTY HEARTY

- Determine what's worthy. Buffets don't have to be all-you-can-eat.
  What looks too good to pass up? What can you live without?
  Focus on what you will enjoy, not on how much you can squeeze
  onto your plate. Decide which items are really "worthy" of splurg-
  ing, and leave the other foods on the table.

- Budget wisely. Balance your calories over the course of the day, or
  at least over the course of a couple of days. If you know that you
  will be consuming extra calories at a social event in the evening,
  try to make adjustments earlier in the day. Focus on fruits and
  veggies, and add some lean protein and high-fiber grains to keep
  your appetite in check. Make healthy and filling choices before-

hand so that you can budget a few more calories to account for the party fare.

- Think before you bite. Think first before you try every irresistible food that crosses your path. How will you feel after you eat that food item? Is the taste really worth it? Could you enjoy just a smaller amount instead?

- Spurn the party snacks. Don't waste your calories mindlessly by munching salty or sugary snack foods. Save them for the big event: dinner and dessert.

- Decorate your plate. Fill half to three-quarters of your plate with colorful raw veggies and fruits or items that have these as their main ingredient, and fill the rest of your plate with lean meat, shrimp or other seafood choices.

- Watch out for calorie culprits. Creamy sauces and cheesy toppings will add extra calories, so take these items in smaller quantities and discretely move some or all to the side of your plate. You will still get the flavor, just not all of the unnecessary calories and fat.

- Plan for indulgence. If you want to indulge in a homemade holiday treat or luscious dessert, ask yourself what you're willing to give up in exchange. Are you willing to give up something at lunch or dinner, or your afternoon snack? Or are you willing to put in the extra time at the gym?

- Downsize it. Cut calories by cutting portion sizes. Cut pies into 10 slices (not 6 to 8), cut brownies and cakes into bite-sized pieces, and bake smaller cookies and mini muffins.

- Use a smaller plate. Make just one trip to the food table and fill only a salad-sized plate with your favorites. This will help you to keep the portion sizes under control.

WHEN THE PARTY'S OVER

- Send the leftovers home with the guests. If you end up with leftovers that are tempting, send them home with your guests or share them with an elderly friend or family member. If you are unable to give all of the leftovers away, freeze some of them in single-serving containers to use for lunches or to have for dinners on the run.

- Purge your pantry. In preparation for the new year, purge your pantry of any junk foods or tempting foods. Out with the old, in with the new!

A NEW BEGINNING

- Write your goals. Are your goals specific and positive? For example, if you have set a goal of exercising more in the upcoming year, instead of just "vowing" to run or work out each day, say something more specific such as "I will run for 15 minutes each day" or "I will work out in the gym for 30 minutes three times each week." Make sure to reword each of your goals so that they are clear and measurable.

- Post your goals. Put your written goals in places where you will see them the most often, such as on your computer, on your refrigerator, in a picture frame on your desk, in a book you are reading, or in your wallet. These reminders will help you to stay focused and on track.

WORRY-FREE THANKSGIVING

- Make desserts the day before. This simple step makes sense and will really help you when it comes time to preparing the Thanksgiving meal. It's often hard to bake everything at the same time, because different items require baking at different temperatures.

- Prepare the day before. Prepare as many food items as possible for the Thanksgiving meal the day before. For instance, you could peel potatoes the day before Thanksgiving and place them in a bowl of water in the refrigerator to keep them from turning brown. When you are ready to cook the potatoes, simply drain the water and cook them as you normally would. You can also make cornbread for homemade dressing and cut up vegetables the day before.

- Buy vegetables that are easy to prepare. Pick up pre-washed bags of salad greens and add baby carrots or grape tomatoes to make a salad in minutes. Buy packages of veggies, such as baby carrots or celery sticks, for quick snacks.

- Zap 'em! Use a microwave to quickly zap vegetables. White or sweet potatoes can be baked quickly this way.

- Accept the help. Whenever anyone offers to help you cook or bring a dish, say, "Yes, thank you!"

- Get creative. Use hollowed bread loaves to make charming serving containers for cheeses, dips, olives, chips and small sandwiches.

- Plan an after-dinner activity. Instead of sitting around after the meal is over and passing around plate after plate of leftovers, plan something for the family to do. Pre-purchase movie tickets for the opening blockbuster and fold them in your napkins. Have your yard staked out for a game of flag football. Your guests will love having the planning done for them!

- Don't sweat it. The secret to being a gracious host (and keeping your own sanity) is to not let small problems ruin the day. If one of your side dishes burns, simply toss it out and enjoy the bounty that you do have. If the turkey burns, order take-out. Don't sweat the small stuff—and don't forget to laugh.

BRINGING JOY TO OTHERS

And let us consider how we may spur one another on toward love and good deeds.
HEBREWS 10:24

- Volunteer and give donations. Volunteer to serve a holiday meal to needy families and give donations to a food pantry. You could even give a gift to someone in another country through organizations such as Samaritan's Purse (see www.samaritanspurse.org).

- Send cards to military service personnel. Visit www.anysoldier.com for more information.

- Send Christmas notes to at least six people who blessed you this past year. For example, you could send a thank-you note to your First Place 4 Health leader or other member in your group who has encouraged you. Be specific as to how they have helped you this year.

- Call someone who may be feeling sad this holiday season. Call a friend who has endured some form of crisis this past year, such as a death in the family this year or an illness, and let that person know you are thinking of him or her.

- Tell stories of family Christmases past. Find old decorations, cards, photos, gifts or other visual reminders of past Christmases that you and your family have experienced. Share stories that you have heard from older relatives about their Christmases. Such heirloom stories tie families to their heritages and encourage them to make memories for the future.

HEALTHY HOLIDAY COOKING TIPS

- Gravies or sauces: If you are making pan gravy, first skim the fat off the pan drippings. For cream or white sauces, use fat-free (skim) milk and soft-tub or liquid margarine.

- Dressings or stuffing: Add low-sodium broth or pan drippings with the fat skimmed off instead of lard or butter. Use herbs and spices and whole grain bread for added flavor.

- Biscuits: Use vegetable oil instead of lard or butter and use fat-free (skim) milk or 1 percent buttermilk instead of regular milk.

- Salads: Use skin-free smoked turkey, liquid smoke, fat-free bacon bits or low-fat bacon instead of fatty meats in the salads.

- Sweet potato pie: Mash sweet potatoes with orange juice concentrate, nutmeg, vanilla, cinnamon and only one egg. Leave out the butter.

- Cakes, cookies, quick breads and pancakes: Use egg whites or an egg substitute instead of whole eggs. Two egg whites can be substituted in many recipes for one whole egg. Use applesauce instead to reduce some of the fat.

- Meats and poultry (chicken and turkey): Trim away all of the visible fat from meats and poultry before cooking. Drain off any fat that appears during cooking.

- Broth: Chill meat and poultry broth until the fat becomes solid, and then skim off fat before using it.

- Breading: Skip or limit the breading on meat, poultry and fish. Breading adds fat and calories, and it will also cause the food to soak up more fat during frying.

STAYING EMOTIONALLY HEALTHY

- Get connected. Call up someone you know or get a group of friends together and plan a night out. Meet for coffee, take a walk on a cool day, or do something you love with someone you care about. Take the initiative. It's common for people to want to wait until someone else reaches out to them—mostly because they want to know that someone cares—but during the holidays you are probably going to have to be the one who makes the initiative to get connected with the other person.

- Rethink your expectations. Rethink what is realistic and base your expectations not on what you *hope* will happen this year but on what you *know* will happen. Don't think about what should be happening, but plan on what has happened in the past. Then you can rejoice if something different occurs!

- Remember to SEE. **S**leep, **E**xercise and **E**at well during the holiday season. It's easy to give up on these three things when you are feeling stressed, depressed or anxious because of the demands of the season. However, if you are intentional about sleeping, exercising and eating well, it will help you to cope better during the holidays.

- Be prepared for family gatherings. If you've never had the perfect Christmas with your family before, don't think that this year will be any different. Be prepared. Make a list of each of the people you will be with on Christmas and how they normally handle the occasion. Think about some of the funny situations you have encountered with your family during past Christmases—remembering and laughing about them now will help you to prepare for what will happen this year. Remember that when you are under stress—as often occurs during the holiday season –your best side won't always show through, so you need to be realistic about what Christmas will be like.

- Be intentional with your time. Think about the amount of time you will spend with your family and friends this year. It's not a bad thing to recognize that you do best spending just a few days together with your family. If you know that you'll be together for a week, plan a trip in the middle of the visit, or take a break each day to do something with the people with whom you do the best.

- Let your faith speak louder than your words. If you have family members who don't share your faith, you might want to try to make the most of every opportunity to share Christ. Sometimes your relatives will perceive this as you coming at them with both guns loaded. Remember that often the best Christmas witness is sharing the life that God has given you. Just talk with your unsaved family members about how blessed you are and show them Christ's love in your life. If they see what you have—Christ, the hope of glory—they will want to have it as well!

- Smile! Grinning, even if you don't feel happy, releases serotonin in the brain, which will instantly lift your mood and make you feel better.

- Start a journal. Use your journal to record positive experiences and things for which you are thankful. Read your past journal entries during times when you feel down to remind yourself how fortunate you truly are.

leader discussion guide

The First Place 4 Health holiday session is six weeks long with one group meeting per week, and is recommended for any member who has completed at least one regular First Place 4 Health session. This shorter session is specially designed for First Place 4 Health members who desire to maintain their healthy habits during the holidays.

Each group meeting should last approximately one hour, with 15-minute segments set aside for (1) weigh-in and memory verse recitation, (2) Wellness Spotlight, (3) devotion/journal discussion, and (4) prayer requests and prayer. Before the first meeting, your group members should memorize the Week One memory verse as they read the daily devotions, complete the journaling assignments, and complete the prayer partner form to turn in during class. They should also fill out their Live It Tracker each day and turn it in at the group meeting. (See the *First Place 4 Health Leader's Guide* for tips on how to evaluate your members' Live It Trackers.)

Following is a suggested outline for each of the six group meetings for this study.

WEEK ONE: VICTORY IN JESUS
Weigh-in and Memory Verse (15 minutes)
Weigh and measure members and listen as they recite the week's Scripture memory verse.

Wellness Spotlight (15 minutes)

Staying motivated during the holidays can be especially difficult, but staying motivated can be difficult at any time of the year if one loses sight of how he or she can benefit from his or her weight-loss efforts. Ask members to share their answers to the following:

1. Have you ever gained weight during the holidays?
2. What tempts you to overeat?
3. What's the payoff when you overeat? What do you get out of overeating?
4. What might you gain by staying focused during this holiday season?

Guide your members to make realistic goals for the holiday session. Have them discuss in small groups or with the whole group some strategies that may keep them focused on their holiday goals.

List these strategies on a whiteboard, chalkboard or poster board. If they have not yet done so, have them complete the goal-making exercise in the introduction of this book.

Devotion/Journal Discussion (15 minutes)

Invite volunteers to share about victories they have experienced and how it helped them to be thankful when they were battle weary.

Ask members to share Scripture verses that have brought comfort or healing to their life.

Prayer Requests/Prayer (15 minutes)

Have members write a praise or something for which they are thankful on small index cards. Send a basket around and fill it with the blessings.

For the prayer time, read the praises, and then ask each member to pray by speaking a one-word praise (e.g., children, health, Jesus).

Before the group leaves, pass around the basket again for prayer partner forms. Have members take a form from the basket on their way out.

WEEK TWO: NO WORRIES
Weigh-in and Memory Verse (15 minutes)
Weigh and measure members and listen as they recite the week's Scripture memory verse.

Wellness Spotlight (15 minutes)
Each of your group members will certainly want to survive the holidays with his or her healthy habits still in place. So, for this session, you will begin to plan activities with your group that will take them through the holidays and enable them to become healthier physically, emotionally, mentally and spiritually in the coming year.

Before the meeting, call members and ask them to bring a day-planner or calendar. During the meeting time, have members split into pairs and review the "Focus and Prioritize" section of Holiday Survival Tips. Ask them to make note of any office parties, mall trips or family gatherings during the holidays on their calendar and brainstorm ways they can stay on track in each of these situations. Next, have them note some fun activities they can place on their calendar that don't involve food, such as walking to see neighborhood decorations, singing holiday carols, attending a play or volunteering. Ask them to note healthy activities that they can write on a specific day of their calendar. (See the "Healthy Activities" section of Holiday Survival Tips for ideas.)

Invite partners to pray for each other during the meeting about the activities they have chosen and keep each other accountable in the coming weeks.

Having your members anticipate challenges or obstacles that they will face on Thanksgiving will allow them time to develop strategies to overcome these challenges. Instruct the members to write out what they plan to eat on Thanksgiving Day. Refer them to the 1,400-calorie Thanksgiving Day menu and to the recipes that follow, as well as to "Worry-Free Thanksgiving" in the Holiday Survival Tips.

Devotion/Journal Discussion (15 minutes)

Ask members if they are more likely to worry than pray and how this week's Scripture Memory Verse helped them conquer worry through prayer and thanksgiving.

Ask volunteers who have memorized Philippians 4:6 to quote it for the group. Then have each member tell how God gave him or her peace and contentment in his or her circumstances.

Prayer Requests/Prayer (15 minutes)

Have each member who is comfortable praying aloud say a short prayer of Thanksgiving for his or her present circumstances that are causing him or her to worry.

Before the group leaves, pass around the basket for prayer partner forms. Have each member draw a form from the basket on his or her way out.

WEEK THREE: NAME ABOVE EVERY NAME
Weigh-in and Memory Verse (15 minutes)

Weigh and measure members and listen as they recite the week's Scripture memory verse.

Wellness Spotlight (15 minutes)

Ask members to consider how focusing on giving to others can help them maintain their fitness goals. Refer them to "Bringing Joy to Others" in the Holiday Survival Tips. Ask members to share other volunteer opportunities they've taken part in during the holiday season. Lead a discussion about how these activities might help to put the focus on Christ and others instead of self. Would members' families support these activities? Why or why not?

Devotion/Journal Discussion (15 minutes)

Share how you were given your name, and then go around the group and ask each member to tell how he or she was named and any special meaning that it might have.

Ask members, "What is your focus during this holiday?" Invite volunteers to share how they (as an individual or as a family) keep their focus on the birth of Christ rather than on buying gifts.

Discuss all of the roles that they take on, such as mom, dad, sister, wife, volunteer, Sunday School teacher, choir member, and so on during this busy season.

As a group, read Isaiah 9:6 aloud, and then list the names of Jesus that are stated in this verse. Ask members which name they need to call on to meet the needs of a specific responsibility that they must fulfill.

Prayer Requests/Prayer (15 minutes)

Invite members to pray aloud short prayers that use the names of Jesus from Isaiah 9:6.

Before the group leaves, pass around the basket for prayer partner forms. Have each member draw a form from the basket on his or her way out.

Note: For next week's meeting, invite volunteers to bring in a holiday party food, such as a dip, finger food or treat, using one of the holiday recipes or one of their own light recipes. If they bring a recipe of their own, ask them to provide copies of the recipe for the other members.

Optional: Have a recipe exchange. Invite members to bring copies of at least one light-eating recipe to share with others.

WEEK FOUR: OUR GREAT GOD
Weigh-in and Memory Verse (15 minutes)
Weigh and measure members and listen as they recite the week's Scripture memory verse.

Wellness Spotlight (15 minutes)
In this session, you will experiment with healthy holiday recipes. Read through "Healthy Holiday Cooking Tips" in Holiday Survival Tips, and ask members to share ideas for lightening up favorite holiday recipes.

Discuss the 1,400-calorie Christmas menu and recipes and how they plan on utilizing this tool as they plan their Christmas menu.

Optional: Allow time for members to exchange their light holiday recipes while tasting the foods that were brought to class.

Devotion/Journal Discussion (15 minutes)
Ask members to share with the group how they keep their focus on Jesus during the stresses of the season.

Brainstorm ways that they can show the greatness of God to their neighbors or to the hard-to-love people in their lives.

Ask someone to share the letter they wrote to God this week telling Him how wonderful He is.

Prayer Requests/Prayer (15 minutes)

Invite members to silently pray for the person on their right before closing in prayer.

Before the group leaves, pass around the basket for prayer partner forms. Have each member draw a form from the basket on his or her way out.

WEEK FIVE: A NEW DIRECTION
Weigh-in and Memory Verse (15 minutes)

Weigh and measure members and listen as they recite the week's Scripture memory verse.

Wellness Spotlight (15 minutes)

In this session, the group will focus on spreading joy to others. Before the meeting, gather blank cards and other supplies (construction paper, stickers, rubber stamps and stamp pads, felt-tip pens, glue, and so forth) to make greeting cards.

If you have a member who is good with crafts, enlist that person's help in showing members how to make a specific type of card—but remember to keep it simple!

Have each member select one person they want to encourage. Have each member send that person a special New Year's card. Invite volunteers to share about their card's recipient and why they chose that person.

Ask members to plan their New Year's Day menu, using the 1,400-calorie New Year's Day menu and recipes.

Devotion/Journal Discussion (15 minutes)

Invite members to share their dreams for the new year by sharing what new thing they would like to accomplish.

Ask members what their long-term and short-term goals are for a healthier life in the new year, and then list these on a whiteboard or a chalkboard.

Prayer Requests/Prayer (15 minutes)

Invite members to share the areas of commitment or situations in which they need God's power to accomplish, and ask a member to pray specifically for that situation.

Before the group leaves, pass around the basket for prayer partner forms. Have each member draw a form from the basket on his or her way out.

WEEK SIX: THE LIGHT OF THE WORLD

Weigh-in and Memory Verse (15 minutes)

Weigh and measure members and listen as they recite the week's Scripture memory verse.

Wellness Spotlight (15 minutes)

The holidays can be full of joy, but they can also bring many stresses. It is important that your group members learn to manage these negative influences in their lives in order to maintain a healthy and balanced life. Reflecting on this holiday season, ask your group what they can do differently next year to avoid emotional traps.

Have members form pairs and share about holiday stressors. If they feel comfortable, ask them to reflect on any particular days or people that caused them to be especially emotional during the holiday season.

As they review "Stay Emotionally Healthy" in the Holiday Survial Tips, ask them to plan for next year by evaluating what they could have done differently. Have partners pray for one another.

Devotion/Journal Discussion

Invite members to share about some old things that they need to get rid of this year (attitudes, habits, possessions, and so forth).

Have members brainstorm plans for a fresh start and ways that they can support one another to remain faithful to their First Place 4 Health commitment.

Challenge members to bring friends to the next orientation meeting to get the new year off to a great start!

Prayer Requests/Prayer (15 minutes)

Invite members to divide into pairs for a time of prayer. Have each partner pray for the other, asking God to bless them in the coming year and to give them strength to put Him first in their lives.

Before the group leaves, pass around the basket for prayer partner forms. Have each member draw a form from the basket on his or her way out.

First Place 4 Health holiday menus & recipes

Each menu plan is based on approximately 1,400 to 1,500 calories per day. All recipe and menu exchanges were determined using the Master-Cook software, a program that accesses a database containing more than 6,000 food items prepared using the United States Department of Agriculture (USDA) publications and information from food manufacturers. As with any nutritional program, MasterCook calculates the nutritional values of the recipes based on ingredients. Nutrition may vary due to how the food is prepared, where the food comes from, soil content, season, ripeness, processing and method of preparation. For these reasons, please use the recipes and menu plans as approximate guides. Consult a physician and/or a registered dietitian before starting a weight-loss program.

For those who need more calories, add the following to the 1,400-calorie plan:

- 1,800 calories: 2 ounce equivalent of meat, 3 ounce equivalent of bread, $^1/_2$ cup vegetable serving, 1 tsp. fat

- 2,000 calories: 2 ounce equivalent of meat, 4 ounce equivalent of bread, $^1/_2$ cup vegetable serving, 3 tsp. fat

- 2,200 calories: 2 ounce equivalent of meat, 5 ounce equivalent of bread, $^1/_2$ cup vegetable serving, $^1/_2$ cup fruit serving, 5 tsp. fat

- 2,400 calories: 2 ounce equivalent of meat, 6 ounce equivalent of bread, 1 cup vegetable serving, $^1/_2$ cup fruit serving, 6 tsp. fat

Thanksgiving Day Menus and Recipes

Note: Recipes for items ***italicized in bold*** are included below.

MENUS

Breakfast

1 ***Morning Surprise Muffin***   ½ cup orange juice

Nutritional Information: 242 calories; 4.4g fat (17% calories from fat); 5.2g protein; 48.2g carbohydrate; 3.4g fiber; 12mg cholesterol; 190mg sodium

Thanksgiving Meal

1 (6 oz.) serving ***Garlic and Rosemary Slow-Roasted Turkey***
½ cup ***Wild Rice Stuffing***
2 tbsp. ***Fresh Cranberry-Orange Relish***

½ cup ***Sweet Potatoes with Meringue***
1 cup fresh green beans
1 serving ***Crustless Pumpkin Pie***

Nutritional Information: 880 calories; 20.4g fat (21% calories from fat); 83.1g protein; 96.9g carbohydrates; 14.5g fiber; 29.2g cholesterol; 590mg sodium

Dinner

1¼ cups ***Green Salad with Apples and Walnut Dressing***

2 wedges ***Turkey Salad with Chutney on Focaccia***

Nutritional Information: 422 calories; 12.3g fat (25% calories from fat); 27.8g protein; 53.5g carbohydrates; 5.3g fiber; 67.4g cholesterol; 932mg sodium

THANKSGIVING RECIPES

Morning Surprise Muffins
1 cup whole-wheat flour
½ cup all-purpose flour
1 cup regular oats
¾ cup packed brown sugar

1 tbsp. wheat bran
2 tsp. baking soda
¼ tsp. salt
1 cup plain fat-free yogurt

1 cup mashed ripe banana (about 2)
1 large egg
1 cup chopped pitted dates
¾ cup chopped walnuts

½ cup chopped dried pineapple
3 tbsp. ground flaxseed (about
  2 tbsp. whole)
nonstick cooking spray

Preheat oven to 350° F. Place 18 muffin cups liners in muffin cups and coat liners with cooking spray. Lightly spoon whole-wheat flour and all-purpose flour into dry measuring cups and level with a knife. Combine whole-wheat flour, all-purpose flour, oats, brown sugar, wheat bran, baking soda and salt in a large bowl and stir with a whisk. Make a well in the center of the mixture. Combine yogurt, banana and egg and add to the flour mixture, stirring just until moist. Fold in dates, walnuts and pineapple. Spoon batter into the prepared muffin cups and sprinkle evenly with flaxseed. Bake at 350° F for 20 minutes or until muffins spring back when touched lightly in center. Remove muffins from pans immediately and cool on a wire rack. Serves 18.

Nutritional Information: 186 calories; 4.4g fat (22% calories from fat); 4.2g protein; 35.2g carbohydrate; 3.4g fiber; 12mg cholesterol; 190mg sodium

Garlic and Rosemary Slow-Roasted Turkey

1 (12 lb.) fresh or frozen turkey,
  thawed
9 garlic cloves, divided
1 tbsp. chopped fresh rosemary
8 tsp. butter, softened

1 tbsp. paprika
1½ tsp. salt
1½ tsp. pepper
3 sprigs fresh rosemary
nonstick cooking spray

Remove and discard giblets and neck from turkey and trim excess fat. Starting at the neck cavity, loosen the skin from the breast and drumsticks by inserting fingers and gently pushing between skin and meat. Mince 3 garlic cloves. Combine minced garlic, chopped rosemary, butter, paprika, salt and pepper in a small bowl. Rub butter mixture under loosened skin of the turkey and rub over breast and drumsticks. Lift wing tips up and over back and tuck under turkey. Place the remaining 6 garlic cloves and rosemary sprigs in the body cavity of the turkey. Tie legs together with kitchen string and let the turkey stand for 1 hour at room temperature. Preheat oven to 500° F. Place turkey, breast side up, on the rack of a roasting pan coated with nonstick cooking spray. Place the rack in a pan and bake at 500° F for 30 minutes. Reduce heat to 250° F and bake for 2 hours or until a thermometer inserted into meaty part of the thigh registers at 165° F. Remove turkey from the oven and cover loosely with foil. Let stand 20 minutes. Discard skin before serving. Serves 12.

Nutritional Information: 355 calories; 8.6g fat (22% calories from fat); 67g protein; 7g carbohydrate; 3g fiber; 229mg cholesterol; 461mg sodium

Wild Rice Stuffing

1½ cups chopped celery
1 cup chopped onion
1 cup uncooked wild rice
2 garlic cloves, minced
4 cups fat-free, less-sodium chicken
    broth
1½ tbsp. chopped fresh sage

1 cup uncooked long-grain brown
    rice
½ cup chopped dried apricots
½ cup chopped pecans, toasted
½ tsp. salt
½ tsp. freshly ground black pepper
nonstick cooking spray

Heat a Dutch oven over medium-high heat. Coat pan with nonstick cooking spray. Add celery, onion, wild rice and garlic to pan, and then sauté for 3 minutes. Stir in broth and sage and bring to a boil. Cover, reduce heat, and simmer 25 minutes. Stir in brown rice and bring to a boil. Cover, reduce heat, and cook for 30 minutes or until liquid is absorbed. Remove from heat and let stand, covered, 10 minutes. Stir in remaining ingredients. Serves 12.

Nutritional Information: 192 calories; 4g fat (19% calories from fat); 5.1g protein; 34.4g carbohydrate; 3.6g fiber; 243mg sodium

Fresh Cranberry-Orange Relish

1 large orange
¼ cup plus 2 tbsp. sugar

2 (10-oz.) packages fresh cranberries

Grate orange rind and place in a food processor. Peel and section orange over the bowl of the food processor. Add orange sections, sugar and cranberries to the processor and process until coarsely chopped. Cover and refrigerate for at least 1 day. Serves 8 (2 tbsp. servings).

Nutritional Information: 20 calories; 0g fat (0% calories from fat); 0g protein; 5.2g carbohydrate; 0.7g fiber; 0mg sodium

Sweet Potatoes with Meringue

4 lbs. orange sweet potatoes
½ tsp. butter
¾ tsp. salt
½ tsp. freshly ground black pepper
1 tsp. minced fresh thyme

4 egg whites
¼ tsp. cream of tartar
½ cup sugar
½ tsp. vanilla extract

Preheat oven to 375° F. Peel sweet potatoes and cut into ¼-inch slices. Butter an 8″ x 8″ pan and arrange slices in layers, sprinkling with salt, pepper and thyme as you go. Cover with aluminum foil and bake potatoes until they are tender when pierced with a fork (approximately 45 to 90 minutes). Bring 1 cup water to a boil in a medium pot over high heat. Reduce heat to maintain a simmer. Put egg whites and cream of tartar in a rimmed metal bowl that is just big enough to fit into pot over water. Set the bowl over the pot and whisk egg whites constantly until they are hot but not cooking (approximately 3 to 5 minutes). Take the egg whites off the heat and beat until firm peaks form. Sprinkle in sugar and vanilla and beat into stiff, shiny peaks. Spread over cooked sweet potatoes. Put under a broiler until nicely browned and serve hot. Serves 10.

Nutritional Information: 155 calories; .5g fat (.03% calories from fat); 3g protein; 35g carbohydrate; 3.3g fiber; 180mg sodium

Crustless Pumpkin Pie

1 egg
2 egg whites
1 (15 oz.) can solid pack pumpkin
sugar substitute, equivalent to ¾ cup
   sugar
½ cup reduced fat biscuit/baking
   mix

1 tsp. vanilla
1 tsp. cinnamon
½ tsp. ground ginger
¼ tsp. ground cloves
1 (12 oz.) can evaporated milk
1 cup reduced-fat whipped topping
nonstick cooking spray

In a large mixing bowl, combine egg, egg whites, pumpkin, sugar substitute, biscuit/baking mix, vanilla, cinnamon, ginger and cloves until smooth. Gradually stir in evaporated milk. Pour mixture onto a 9-inch pie plate coated with a nonstick cooking spray. Bake at 350° F for 35 to 40 minutes, or until a knife inserted near the center comes out clean. Cool on a wire rack. Dollop with whipped topping before serving. Refrigerate leftovers. Serves 8.

Nutritional Information: 124 calories; 2g fat (15% calories from fat); 6g protein; 19g carbohydrate; 3g fiber; 28mg cholesterol; 160mg sodium

Green Salad with Apples and Walnut Dressing

6 cups gourmet salad greens
1 cup (2-inch) julienne-cut Braeburn apples
2 tbsp. cider vinegar
2 tbsp. maple syrup

2 tsp. Dijon mustard
1½ tsp. walnut oil
$^1/_8$ tsp. salt
$^1/_8$ tsp. ground red pepper

Combine salad greens and Braeburn apple in a large bowl. Combine vinegar, syrup, Dijon mustard, walnut oil, salt and ground red pepper, stirring with a whisk. Drizzle over salad and toss gently to coat. Serves 4.

Nutritional Information: 73 calories; 2.2g fat (28% calories from fat); 1.6g protein; 13.7g carbohydrate; 2.5g fiber; 0mg cholesterol; 159mg sodium

Turkey Salad with Chutney on Focaccia

½ cup finely chopped celery
$^1/_3$ cup hot mango chutney
3 tbsp. light mayonnaise
1 tsp. sesame seeds, toasted
2 cups (10 oz.) chopped cooked turkey
1 (5¼ oz.) package focaccia (Italian flatbread) or 2 (6-inch) pitas
8 spinach leaves

1 small zucchini, cut lengthwise into 8 (¼-inch) slices
1 (7 oz.) bottle roasted red bell peppers, drained and sliced
2 tbsp. reduced-fat Caesar dressing
4 tsp. Dijon mustard
olive oil-flavored cooking spray

Preheat oven to 350° F. Combine celery, chutney, mayonnaise and sesame seeds in a medium bowl. Add turkey and toss gently to coat. Cut each bread piece in half horizontally and spray the cut sides of each piece with olive-oil flavored cooking spray. Place bread slices in a single layer on a jelly-roll pan. Bake at 350° F for 12 minutes or until toasted. Spread ½ cup of the turkey salad over each bottom half and top with zucchini slices, roasted peppers and spinach. Drizzle with dressing. Spread mustard over the top halves of bread and place on top of the sandwiches. Cut each sandwich into 4 wedges. Serves 4.

Nutritional Information: 349 calories; 10.1g fat (26% calories from fat); 26.2g protein; 38.6g carbohydrates; 2.8g fiber; 65mg cholesterol; 733mg sodium

ADDITIONAL THANKSGIVING RECIPES

Open-Faced Turkey Sandwich with Apple and Cheese

4 (2 oz.) slices country or peasant
bread
4 tsp. low-fat mayonnaise
4 tsp. Dijon mustard
1 cup trimmed arugula
4 ($^1/_8$-inch-thick) slices red onion
12 oz. thinly sliced deli turkey

2 Pink Lady or Cameo apples, cored
and cut crosswise into 8 (¼-inch-
thick) slices
½ cup (2 oz.) grated Havarti cheese
coarsely ground black pepper (optional)

Preheat a broiler with the oven rack in the middle position. Spread each bread slice with 1 tsp. mayonnaise and 1 tsp. mustard. Layer each slice with ¼ cup arugula, 1 onion slice, 3 oz. turkey, 4 apple slices and 2 tbsp. cheese. Place the sandwiches on a baking sheet and broil 4 minutes, or until cheese is bubbly. Remove from heat and sprinkle with pepper (if desired). Serve immediately. Serves 4.

Nutritional Information: 427 calories; 14.1g fat (30% calories from fat); 29.9g protein; 44.2g carbohydrate; 5.7g fiber; 69mg cholesterol; 634mg sodium

Turkey and Wild Rice Salad

1 cup uncooked wild rice blend
$^1/_3$ cup leftover whole-berry cranberry sauce
2 tbsp. turkey stock
1½ tbsp. balsamic vinegar
½ tsp. salt
¼ tsp. freshly ground black pepper
¼ tsp. Dijon mustard

1½ tbsp. extra virgin olive oil
1½ cups shredded cooked turkey
(light and dark meat)
½ cup diced celery
½ cup chopped fresh chives
$^1/_3$ cup dried cranberries
¼ cup chopped fresh parsley
2 cups trimmed watercress

Cook wild rice according to the package directions, omitting salt and fat. Cool. Combine cranberry sauce, turkey stock, vinegar, salt, pepper and mustard in a small bowl. Gradually add the oil, stirring constantly with a whisk. Add cranberry sauce mixture, turkey, celery, chives, cranberries and parsley to the rice mixture and toss gently to coat. Serve over watercress. Serves 4.

Nutritional Information: 261 calories; 8.3g fat (29% calories from fat); 17.7g protein; 28.5g carbohydrate; 1.7g fiber; 41mg cholesterol; 557mg sodium

Spicy Pickled Green Beans

2 cups water
2 cups white vinegar
3 tbsp. kosher salt
1½ tbsp. sugar
8 fresh dill sprigs

3 tbsp. thinly sliced garlic (about 8
  cloves)
4 small dried hot red chiles
1½ lbs. green beans, trimmed

Combine water, vinegar, salt and sugar in a large saucepan and bring to a boil. Remove from heat and add garlic, dill and peppers to the pan. Let stand for 1 minute. Pour vinegar mixture over the beans in a large glass bowl. Cover and refrigerate 1 week, stirring occasionally. Serves 26.

Nutritional Information: 10 calories; 0.1g fat (.09% calories from fat); 0.6g protein; 2.4g carbohydrate; 0.9g fiber; 0mg cholesterol; 120mg sodium

Christmas Day Menus and Recipes

Note: Recipes for items *italicized in bold* are included below.

MENUS

Breakfast

Sausage and Cheese Breakfast Casserole

1 cup orange juice

Nutritional Information: 305 calories; 7.3g fat (22% calories from fat); 17.8g protein; 42g carbohydrate; 1.1g fiber; 76mg cholesterol; 639mg sodium

Lunch

1 cup serving *Spinach Salad with Nectarines and Spicy Pecans*

1 (3 oz.) serving *Garlic and Herb Standing Rib Roast*

½ cup *Roasted Garlic Mashed Potatoes*

½ cup *Broccoli with Lemon Crumbs*

1 slice (1/16 of cake) *Peppermint Ice Cream Cake*

Nutritional Information: 731 calories; 27.2g fat (34% calories from fat); 38.3g protein; 69.6g carbohydrate; 11.1g fiber; 94g cholesterol; 1,041mg sodium

Dinner

1 cup *Spicy Tomato and White Bean Soup*

1 *Extreme Grilled Cheese Sandwich*

Nutritional Information: 533 calories; 15.3g fat (26% calories from fat); 28.3g protein; 73.4g carbohydrate; 10g fiber; 24mg cholesterol; 1,704mg sodium

CHRISTMAS RECIPES

Sausage and Cheese Breakfast Casserole

12 oz. turkey breakfast sausage
2 cups 1% lowfat milk
2 cups egg substitute
1 tsp. dry mustard

¾ tsp. salt
½ tsp. freshly ground black pepper
¼ tsp. ground red pepper
3 large eggs

16 (1 oz.) slices white bread
¼ tsp. paprika
nonstick cooking spray

1 cup (4 oz.) finely shredded
reduced-fat extra sharp
cheddar cheese

Heat a large nonstick skillet over medium-high heat. Coat pan with non-stick cooking spray. Add sausage to pan and cook for 5 minutes or until browned, stirring and breaking sausage to crumble. Remove from heat and cool. Combine milk, egg substitute, mustard, salt, black pepper, red pepper and eggs in a large bowl, stirring with a whisk. Trim crusts from bread. Cut bread into 1-inch cubes and add bread cubes, sausage and cheddar cheese to milk mixture, stirring to combine. Pour bread mixture into a 13" x 9" baking dish or a three quart casserole dish coated with nonstick cooking spray. Spread egg mixture evenly in baking dish. Cover and refrigerate 8 hours or overnight. Preheat oven to 350° F. Remove casserole from refrigerator and let stand for 30 minutes. Sprinkle paprika evenly over the casserole. Bake at 350° F for 45 minutes or until set and lightly browned. Let stand for 10 minutes. Serves 12.

Nutritional Information: 184 calories; 6.8g fat (33% calories from fat); 15.9g protein; 14g carbohydrate; 0.6g fiber; 76mg cholesterol; 636mg sodium

Spinach Salad with Nectarines and Spicy Pecans

¼ cup powdered sugar
½ tsp. salt
¼ tsp. ground allspice
$1/_8$ tsp. ground nutmeg

$1/_8$ tsp. ground red pepper
$1/_3$ cup pecan halves
nonstick cooking spray

Vinaigrette

3 tbsp. finely chopped shallots
3 tbsp. balsamic vinegar
1 tsp. sugar
2 tsp. fresh lemon juice

2 tsp. extra-virgin olive oil
1 tsp. Dijon mustard
¾ tsp. salt
½ tsp. freshly ground black pepper

Salad

¾ cup very thin slices prosciutto, coarsely chopped (about 2 oz.)
2 (6 oz.) packages fresh baby spinach (about 12 cups)

2 nectarines, cut into ¼-inch wedges (about ¾ lb.)

Preheat oven to 350° F. To prepare pecans, first combine powdered sugar, salt, allspice, nutmeg and red pepper in a small bowl. Rinse pecans with cold water and drain—do not allow the pecans to dry. Add pecans to the sugar mixture and toss well to coat. Arrange the pecan mixture on a jelly-roll pan coated with nonstick cooking spray. Bake at 350° F for 10 minutes, stirring occasionally. Coarsely chop pecans and set aside. To prepare vinaigrette, combine the shallots, balsamic vinegar, sugar, lemon juice, extra-virgin olive oil, Dijon mustard, salt and black pepper in a small bowl, stirring with a whisk until blended. To prepare salad, heat a large nonstick skillet coated with nonstick cooking spray over medium-high heat. Add prosciutto and sauté for 5 minutes or until crisp. Chop finely. Combine spinach, nectarines and dressing in a large bowl and toss gently to coat. Sprinkle with the pecans and prosciutto. Serves 12.

Nutritional Information: 75 calories; 4g fat (45% calories from fat); 2.7g protein; 8.2g carbohydrate; 1.5g fiber; 4mg cholesterol; 369mg sodium

Garlic and Herb Standing Rib Roast

1 (5 lb.) standing rib roast, trimmed	4 garlic cloves, minced
1½ tbsp. chopped fresh thyme	parsley sprigs (optional)
½ tsp. salt	roasted garlic heads (optional)
¼ tsp. freshly ground black pepper	nonstick cooking spray

Preheat oven to 450° F. Place the roast on a broiler pan coated with nonstick cooking spray. Combine thyme, salt, pepper and garlic cloves and rub over the roast. Bake at 450° F for 45 minutes. Reduce heat to 350° F (do not remove roast from oven) and bake for 1 hour and 20 minutes or until a thermometer registers 145° F (medium-rare) or desired degree of doneness. Let stand for 10 minutes before slicing. Garnish with parsley and roasted garlic, if desired. Serves 12.

Nutritional Information: 226 calories; 13.3g fat (53% calories from fat); 24.4g protein; 0.4g carbohydrate; 0.1g fiber; 72mg cholesterol; 162mg sodium

Roasted Garlic Mashed Potatoes

1 garlic head	3 cups water
1 tbsp. olive oil	½ cup 1% lowfat milk
1 lb. peeled Yukon Gold or red potatoes, quartered	¼ tsp. salt
	¼ tsp. pepper

Preheat oven to 375° F. Remove white papery skin from garlic head (do not peel or separate cloves). Rub oil over the garlic head and wrap in foil. Bake at 375° F for 1 hour and then cool for 10 minutes. Separate the cloves and squeeze to extract garlic pulp. Set aside and discard skins. Place the potatoes in a saucepan and cover with water. Bring to a boil and cook for 15 minutes or until very tender. Drain the water from the potatoes. Heat the lowfat milk in a pan over medium heat until hot (do not boil). Add potatoes, salt and pepper, and then beat at medium speed of a mixer until potato mixture is smooth. Add garlic pulp, and stir well. Serves 5 (½ cup servings).

Nutritional Information: 105 calories; 3.1g fat (26% calories from fat); 3.9g protein; 16.6g carbohydrate; 1.8g fiber; 140mg sodium

Broccoli with Lemon Crumbs

2 slices whole-wheat bread
2 tbsp. butter
1 lemon
½ tsp. kosher salt

freshly ground black pepper
2 (12 oz.) bags broccoli florets,
    or 1 large bunch broccoli, cut
    into florets

Whirl the bread in a food processor or blender to make into bread crumbs. Melt the butter in a small skillet. Add the bread crumbs and sauté over medium heat until toasted. Grate the zest from the lemon, and then cut the lemon in half and squeeze the juice from one half into the pan. Add the salt and several grinds of black pepper and cook, stirring constantly, until dry. (*Note*: the lemon crumbs can be made up to 2 days ahead. Spoon the lemon crumbs into a plastic bag and set aside at room temperature.) Microwave the broccoli according to the package directions. (If using fresh broccoli, pile the florets on a microwave-safe plate and sprinkle with a few tablespoons of water. Cover with plastic wrap and microwave 3 to 5 minutes or until crisp-tender.) Remove and sprinkle with the lemon crumbs. Serves 10.

Nutritional Information: 34 calories; 0g fat (0% calories from fat); 3mg protein; 6g fiber; 2g cholesterol; 163mg sodium

Peppermint Ice Cream Cake

¾ cup unsweetened cocoa
¾ cup boiling water
6 tbsp. butter, melted

1 cup packed dark brown sugar
½ cup granulated sugar
¾ cup egg substitute

¾ cup unsweetened cocoa
¾ cup boiling water
6 tbsp. butter, melted

1 cup packed dark brown sugar
½ cup granulated sugar
¾ cup egg substitute

Preheat oven to 350° F. Coat 2 (8-inch) round cake pans with cooking spray. Line the bottom of each pan with wax paper. Combine cocoa, water and butter, stirring with a whisk until blended, and then cool. Combine brown sugar and granulated sugar in a large bowl, stirring well until blended. Add egg substitute and beat for 2 minutes or until light and creamy. Add cocoa mixture, and then beat for 1 minute. Lightly spoon flour into dry measuring cups and level with a knife. Combine flour, baking powder, baking soda and salt. Gradually add the flour mixture to bowl, and then beat for 1 minute or until blended. Stir in vanilla. Pour batter into prepared pans and bake at 350° F for 28 minutes or until a wooden pick inserted in center comes out clean. Cool the pans for 10 minutes on a wire rack. Remove the cake from the pans, wrap in plastic wrap, and freeze for 2 hours or until slightly frozen. Next, spread the ice cream in an 8″ round cake pan lined with plastic wrap. Cover and freeze for 4 hours or until firm. To assemble cake, place one cake layer, bottom side up, on a cake pedestal. Remove the ice cream layer from freezer and remove the plastic wrap. Place the ice cream layer, bottom side up, on top of cake layer, and then top with the remaining cake layer. Combine whipped topping and peppermint extract and stir until blended. Spread frosting over the top and sides of the cake. Sprinkle with crushed peppermints and freeze until ready to serve. Let cake stand at room temperature for 10 minutes before slicing. Serves 16.

Nutritional Information: 251 calories; 6.8g fat (24% calories from fat); 4.3g protein; 44.4g carbohydrate; 1.7g fiber; 19mg cholesterol; 207mg sodium

Spicy Tomato and White Bean Soup

1 (14 oz.) can fat-free, less-sodium chicken broth, divided
2 tsp. chili powder
1 tsp. ground cumin
1 (16 oz.) can navy beans, drained and rinsed
1 medium poblano chile, halved and seeded

½ onion, cut into ½-inch-thick wedges
1 pint grape tomatoes
¼ cup chopped fresh cilantro
2 tbsp. fresh lime juice
1 tbsp. extra-virgin olive oil
½ tsp. salt
cilantro sprigs (optional)

Combine 1 cup broth, chili powder, cumin and beans in a Dutch oven over medium-high heat. Combine the remaining broth, chile and onion in a food processor and pulse until vegetables are chopped. Add onion mixture to pan. Add the tomatoes and cilantro to food processor and process until coarsely chopped. Add tomato mixture to pan and bring to a boil. Cover, reduce heat and simmer 5 minutes or until vegetables are tender. Remove from the heat and stir in juice, olive oil and salt. Garnish with cilantro sprigs, if desired. Serves 4.

Nutritional Information: 157 calories; 4.3g fat (25% calories from fat); 8.1g protein; 23.1g carbohydrate; 6.7g fiber; 0mg cholesterol; 828mg sodium

Extreme Grilled Cheese Sandwich

1 cup vertically sliced red onion
1 large garlic clove, minced
1 cup (4 oz.) shredded reduced-fat sharp white cheddar cheese (such as Cracker Barrel)
2 cups fresh spinach leaves

8 (1½ oz.) slices hearty white bread (such as Pepperidge Farm)
8 (¼-inch-thick) tomato slices
6 slices center-cut bacon, cooked
nonstick cooking spray

Heat a large nonstick skillet over medium-low heat. Coat pan with nonstick cooking spray. Add 1 cup onion and garlic. Cook for 10 minutes or until tender and golden brown, stirring occasionally. Sprinkle 2 tbsp. cheese over each of 4 bread slices. Top each slice with ½ cup spinach, 2 tomato slices, 2 tbsp. of the onion mixture, and 1½ bacon slices. Sprinkle each sandwich with 2 tbsp. cheese, and then top with the remaining 4 bread slices. Heat skillet over medium heat. Coat pan with nonstick cooking spray. Place sandwiches in pan and cook for 3 minutes on each side or until golden brown and cheese melts. Serves 4.

Nutritional Information: 376 calories; 11g fat (26% calories from fat); 20.2g protein; 50.3g carbohydrate; 3.3g fiber; 24mg cholesterol; 876mg sodium

ADDITIONAL CHRISTMAS RECIPES

Sugar-Free Cocoa Mix

2⅓ cups instant nonfat dry milk
⅓ cup unsweetened cocoa
⅓ cup granulate calorie-free sweetener

miniature marshmallows (optional)
sugar-free candy canes (optional)

Combine nonfat dry milk, unsweetened cocoa and calorie-free sweetener in a large bowl and stir well. Store in an airtight container. To serve, spoon ¼ cup of the cocoa mix into each mug. Add 1 cup boiling water and stir well. Top with miniature marshmallows or sugar-free candy canes, if desired (note that marshmallows and candy canes are not included in the nutritional information below). Serves 12.

Nutritional Information: 62 calories; 0.4g fat (0.07% calories from fat); 5.1g protein; 13.5g carbohydrate; 0.8g fiber; 2mg cholesterol; 73mg sodium

Hash Brown Casserole with Bacon, Onions and Cheese

6 bacon slices
1 cup chopped onion
2 garlic cloves, minced
1 (32 oz.) package frozen Southern-
  style hash brown potatoes
1 cup (4 oz.) shredded four-cheese
  blend, divided
½ cup chopped green onions
½ cup fat-free sour cream

½ tsp. salt
¼ tsp. freshly ground black pepper
1 (10.75 oz.) can 30% reduced
  sodium, 98% fat-free condensed
  cream of mushroom soup,
  undiluted
nonstick cooking spray

Cook bacon in a large nonstick skillet over medium heat until crisp. Remove bacon from pan and crumble. Discard drippings from pan. Add 1 cup onion and garlic to the pan and cook for 5 minutes or until tender, stirring frequently. Stir in the potatoes, and then cover and cook for 15 minutes, stirring occasionally. Combine the crumbled bacon, ¼ cup cheese, green onions, sour cream, salt, pepper and soup in a large bowl. Add the potato mixture and toss gently to combine. Spoon mixture into an 11" x 7" baking dish coated with nonstick cooking spray and sprinkle with the remaining ¾ cup cheese. Cover with foil coated with nonstick cooking spray. Refrigerate for 8 hours or overnight. Preheat oven to 350° F. Remove casserole from refrigerator and let stand at room temperature 15 minutes. Bake the casserole, covered, at 350° F for 30 minutes. Uncover and bake an additional 30 minutes or until bubbly around edges and the cheese begins to brown. Serves 6.

Nutritional Information: 293 calories; 10g fat (31% calories from fat); 12.2g protein; 41.4g carbohydrate; 4.7g fiber; 31mg cholesterol; 720mg sodium

Carrots Roasted with Spanish Paprika

2 tbsp. olive oil
1½ tsp. Spanish smoked paprika
1 tsp. kosher salt
½ tsp. freshly ground black pepper

2½ lbs. medium carrots, peeled and
  halved lengthwise
2 tbsp. finely chopped fresh cilantro

Place a jellyroll pan on bottom oven rack. Preheat oven to 450° F. Combine olive oil, paprika, salt, pepper and carrots in a large bowl and toss well. Arrange carrot mixture in a single layer on a preheated pan. Bake at 450° F for 25 minutes or until tender, stirring after 12 minutes. Sprinkle with cilantro. Serves 4.

Nutritional Information: 72 calories; 3g fat (38% calories from fat); 0.1g protein; 11.1g carbohydrate; 3.3g fiber; 0mg cholesterol; 267mg sodium

Lemon Drop Cookies

½ cup granulated sugar
7 tbsp. butter or stick margarine,
  softened
2 tsp. grated lemon rind
⅓ cup honey
½ tsp. lemon extract
1 large egg
1¾ cups all-purpose flour

1 tsp. baking powder
½ tsp. salt
¼ cup plain fat-free yogurt
1 cup powdered sugar
2 tbsp. fresh lemon juice
2 tsp. grated lemon rind
nonstick cooking spray

Preheat oven to 350° F. Beat first 3 ingredients with a mixer at medium speed until light and fluffy. Add honey, extract and egg and beat until well blended. Lightly spoon flour into dry measuring cups and level with a knife. Combine flour, baking powder and salt, stirring well with a whisk. Add flour mixture to sugar mixture alternately with yogurt, beginning and ending with the flour mixture. Drop the mixture by level tablespoons 2 inches apart onto baking sheets coated with nonstick cooking spray. Bake at 350° F for 12 minutes or until lightly browned. Combine powdered sugar and juice in a small bowl and stir with a whisk. Brush powdered sugar mixture evenly over the hot cookies and sprinkle evenly with 2 tsp. rind. Remove the cookies from the pan and cool on wire racks. Makes 32 cookies.

Nutritional Information: 89 calories; 2.8g fat (29% calories from fat); 1.1g protein; 15.3g carbohydrate; 0.2g fiber; 14mg cholesterol; 81mg sodium

Ginger Cookies

6 tbsp. butter, softened
$^2/_3$ cup plus 3 tbsp. sugar, divided
¼ cup molasses
1 large egg
2 cups all-purpose flour (about 9 oz.)

2 tsp. baking soda
1 tsp. ground ginger
1 tsp. ground cinnamon
½ tsp. ground mace
nonstick cooking spray

Place butter in a large bowl and beat with a mixer at medium speed until fluffy. Gradually add $^2/_3$ cup sugar, beating at medium speed until light and well blended. Add molasses and egg and beat well. Lightly spoon flour into dry measuring cups and level with a knife. Combine flour, baking soda, ginger, cinnamon and mace, stirring with a whisk. Gradually add the flour mixture to the butter mixture, stirring until well blended. Divide the dough in half. Wrap each portion in plastic wrap and freeze for 30 minutes. Next, preheat oven to 350° F. Shape each portion of dough into 26 (1-inch) balls. Roll the balls in the remaining 3 tbsp. sugar and place 2 inches apart on baking sheets coated with nonstick cooking spray. Flatten the cookies with the bottom of a glass to ½-inch thickness. Bake at 350° F for 12 minutes or until lightly browned. Remove from pans and cool completely on wire racks. Makes 52 cookies.

Nutritional Information: 48 calories; 1.5g fat (31% calories from fat); 0.6g protein; 8.2g carbohydrate; 0.2g fiber; 8mg cholesterol; 60mg sodium

New Year's Day Menus and Recipes

Note: Recipes for items *italicized in bold* are included below.

MENUS

Breakfast

2 slices whole-wheat toast
½ tbsp. light margarine

1 (6 oz.) lowfat yogurt
½ cup berries

Nutritional Information: 253 calories; 3g fat (11% calories from fat), 15g protein; 44g carbohydrate; 5g fiber; 3mg cholesterol; 426mg sodium

Lunch

1 *Turkey Reuben Panini*
1 cup *Tortilla Soup with Roasted Tomatoes*
1 cup fresh fruit

Nutritional Information: 463 calories; 14.3g fat (28% calories from fat); 32g protein; 53.1g carbohydrates; 10.8g fiber; 44g cholesterol; 714mg sodium

Dinner

Mixed Green Salad
Spicy Chicken with Black-Eyed Peas and Rice

½ cup lowfat, no-sugar-added ice cream with 2 tbsp. Hershey's syrup and 2 tbsp. Cool Whip Lite®

Nutritional Information: 629 calories; 6.5g fat (9% calories from fat); 56.5g protein; 92g carbohydrates; 17g fiber; 99g cholesterol; 22.5mg sodium

NEW YEAR'S RECIPES

Turkey Reuben Panini
8 (½ oz.) slices thin-sliced
  rye bread

¼ cup fat-free Thousand Island
  dressing

8 (½ oz.) thin slices reduced-fat Swiss cheese

¼ cup refrigerated sauerkraut, rinsed and drained

8 oz. deli low-sodium turkey breast (such as Boar's Head®)

Spread all pieces of bread slices evenly with 1½ tsp. dressing. Place one cheese slice on dressed side of each slice and top each with 1 tbsp. sauerkraut and 2 oz. turkey. Top each sandwich with 1 cheese slice and 1 bread slice, dressed side down. Coat the outside of the sandwich (top and bottom) with cooking spray. Heat a large skillet over medium-high heat and add sandwiches to the pan. Place a cast-iron or other heavy skillet on top of sandwiches and press gently to flatten sandwiches (leave the cast-iron skillet on the sandwiches while they cook). Cook 2 minutes on each side or until browned and cheese melts. Serves 4.

Nutritional Information: 268 calories; 7.5g fat (25% calories from fat); 25.3g protein; 25.7g carbohydrate; 3.1g fiber; 35mg cholesterol; 819mg sodium

Tortilla Soup with Roasted Tomato

5 medium tomatoes, cut in half (about 1½ lbs.)

2 (6-inch) Anaheim chiles

7 (¼-inch-thick) slices onion

2 large garlic cloves, halved

8 (6-inch) white corn tortillas, cut into ½-inch strips

1 tbsp. chopped fresh cilantro

2 tsp. ground cumin

½ tsp. sugar

½ tsp. salt

¼ tsp. freshly ground black pepper

3 (14 oz.) cans fat-free, less-sodium chicken broth

½ cup diced ripe avocado

½ cup (2 oz.) shredded queso fresco

8 cilantro sprigs

nonstick cooking spray

Preheat broiler. Arrange tomatoes, cut sides down, on a foil-lined baking sheet. Cut chiles in half lengthwise and discard seeds and membranes. Place chiles, skin sides up, on baking sheet and flatten with hand. Broil for 15 minutes or until blackened, and then remove from the oven and let stand 15 minutes. Peel the tomatoes and chiles and place in a small bowl. Place the onion and garlic on a baking sheet. Lightly coat with cooking spray and broil 20 minutes or until browned, turning after 10 minutes. Add onion and garlic to the tomatoes in a bowl. Discard the foil. Arrange tortilla strips in a single layer on a baking sheet and coat with nonstick cooking spray. Broil for 9 minutes or until lightly browned, stirring occasionally. Place the tomatoes, chiles, onion and garlic in a food processor and process for 1 minute or until blended. Spoon the tomato mixture into a large saucepan and cook over medium heat 2 minutes, stirring constantly. Reduce heat to low and cook for another 6 minutes, stirring occasionally. Stir in the cilantro, cumin, sugar, salt, pepper and chicken broth and bring to a boil. Cover, reduce heat and simmer for another 15 minutes. Ladle 1 cup of the soup into each of 8 bowls, and then top each serving with 6 tortilla strips, 1 tbsp. avocado, 1 tbsp. queso fresco and 1 cilantro sprig. Serves 8.

Nutritional Information: 149 calories; 6.8g fat (41% calories from fat), 5.8g protein; 17.5g carbohydrate; 4.6g fiber; 9mg cholesterol; 490mg sodium

Spicy Chicken with Black-Eyed Peas and Rice

1 tbsp. olive oil, divided
1 tsp. paprika
1 tsp. Old Bay seasoning
½ tsp. sugar
¼ tsp. salt
4 (6 oz.) skinless, boneless chicken breast halves
1 cup chopped onion

1 tsp. bottled minced garlic
1½ cups cooked long-grain rice
1 tsp. hot pepper sauce (such as Tabasco®)
1 (15.8 oz.) can black-eyed peas, undrained
¼ cup sliced green onions

Preheat oven to 350° F. Heat 2 tsp. of oil in a large nonstick skillet over medium heat. In a small bowl, combine paprika, seasoning, sugar and ¼ tsp. salt. Sprinkle over the chicken. Add the chicken to the pan and cook 2 minutes on each side. Wrap the handle of the pan with foil and place the pan in oven. Bake at 350° F for 6 minutes or until chicken is done. Cover and keep warm. Heat 1 tsp. of the oil in a large saucepan over medium heat. Add onion and garlic and sauté 3 minutes. Stir in rice, ¼ tsp. salt, hot pepper sauce and black-eyed peas. Cook for 3 minutes or until thoroughly heated, stirring frequently. Spoon about ¾ cup of the rice mixture into each of 4 bowls and top each serving with 1 chicken breast half. Sprinkle with 1 tbsp. green onions. Serves 4.

Nutritional Information: 405 calories; 6.5g fat (15% calories from fat); 47g protein; 37.5g carbohydrate; 5g fiber; 99mg cholesterol; 868mg sodium

ADDITIONAL NEW YEAR'S RECIPES

Black Bean Dip with Lime

2 (15 oz.) cans black beans, rinsed and drained
1 cup grated carrot
½ cup fresh lime juice (about 2 limes)
¼ cup finely chopped green onions
¼ cup chopped fresh cilantro
1 tsp. minced garlic
¼ tsp. salt
$1/_8$ tsp. ground red pepper
baked tortilla chips

Place beans in a food processor and pulse until almost smooth. Combine the beans, carrot, lime juice, onions, cilantro, garlic, salt and red pepper in a medium bowl, stirring until well blended. Let stand for 30 minutes. Serve with baked tortilla chips. Makes 5 cups.

Nutritional Information: 19 calories; 0.1g fat (0.05% calories from fat); 1.2g protein; 3.9g carbohydrate; 1.3g fiber; 0mg cholesterol; 61mg sodium

Creamy Corn and Chorizo-Stuffed Mushrooms

6 oz. Mexican chorizo sausage (or any ground sausage)
½ cup finely chopped onion
2 garlic cloves, minced
1 (11 oz.) can extra sweet whole-kernel corn, drained
2 oz. $1/_3$-less-fat cream cheese
¼ cup fat-free sour cream
½ tsp. salt
2 (1 oz.) slices white bread
24 stuffer mushroom caps (or large mushrooms with stems removed)
nonstick cooking spray

Preheat oven to 400° F. To prepare the stuffing, remove casings from the chorizo. Cook chorizo, onion and garlic in a large nonstick skillet over medium heat for 6 minutes or until browned, stirring to crumble. Drain the chorizo mixture and pat dry with paper towels. Combine chorizo mixture and corn in a bowl. Combine cream cheese and sour cream in a small bowl and stir with a whisk until smooth. Add the cheese mixture and salt to the chorizo mixture. Place white bread in a food processor and pulse 10 times or until fine crumbs measure 1 cup. Fill each mushroom cap with about ¾ tsp. breadcrumbs. Stuff each with 2 tsp. corn mixture and top with remaining breadcrumbs. Place the mushrooms on a baking sheet coated with nonstick cooking spray. Coat each mushroom with nonstick cooking spray and bake at 400° F for 20 minutes or until tops are browned. Makes 12 servings (2 mushroom serving size).

Nutritional Information: 105 calories; 5.6g fat (49% calories from fat); 5.7g protein; 9.1g carbohydrate; 1.1g fiber; 13mg cholesterol; 325mg sodium

Vegetarian Stuffed Peppers

6 medium red or green bell peppers
1 tsp. olive oil
¾ cup finely chopped shallots
4 cups chopped mushrooms
1 cup chopped fresh parsley
¼ cup slivered almonds, toasted
3 tbsp. dry sherry

1½ tsp. ancho chile powder
2½ cups hot cooked brown rice
1 cup tomato juice
½ tsp. freshly ground black pepper
½ tsp. garlic powder
¼ tsp. salt
¼ cup (1 oz.) grated Parmesan cheese

Preheat oven to 350° F. Cut the tops off of the bell peppers and discard seeds and membranes. Cook peppers in boiling water for 5 minutes and drain. Heat oil in a large nonstick skillet over medium-high heat. Add shallots and sauté for 3 minutes or until tender. Add mushrooms and sauté for 4 minutes or until tender. Add parsley, almonds, sherry and chile powder and sauté for 3 minutes. Add rice, tomato juice, black pepper, garlic powder and salt and sauté for 3 minutes. Spoon ¾ cup of the rice mixture into each bell pepper. Top each bell pepper with 2 tsp. cheese. Place the stuffed bell peppers in a 13″ x 9″ baking dish. Bake at 350° F for 15 minutes. Serves 6.

Nutritional Information. 234 calories; 5.9g fat (23% calories from fat); 84g protein; 39.2g carbohydrate; 6.7g fiber; 3mg cholesterol; 402mg sodium

Warm Caramelized-Onion Dip

2 tsp. olive oil
4 cups chopped onion (about 2 large onions)
¾ tsp. chopped fresh thyme
½ cup light sour cream
$1/3$ cup grated Parmigiano-Reggiano cheese (about 1½ oz.)

$1/3$ cup (3 oz.) $1/3$ less-fat cream cheese
$1/3$ cup reduced-fat mayonnaise
¼ tsp. salt
¼ tsp. freshly ground black pepper
¼ tsp. hot pepper sauce (such as Tabasco®)
¼ tsp. Worcestershire sauce

Heat the olive oil in a large, nonstick skillet over medium-high heat, swirling to coat the pan. Add chopped onion and thyme to the pan and sauté 10 minutes or until golden brown. Reduce heat to low and cook for 20 minutes or until onions are deep golden brown, stirring occasionally. Remove the onion mixture from heat. Add sour cream and the remaining ingredients, stirring until blended and the cheese melts. Serve with whole-grain crackers or baked chips. Serves 12 (3 tbsp. serving size).

Nutritional Information: 81 calories; 4.9g fat (55% calories from fat); 3.1g protein; 7.7g carbohydrate; 0.9g fiber; 12mg cholesterol; 206mg sodium

Black-Eyed Peas and Seafood Salad

3 bacon slices
¾ cup finely chopped celery
1/3 cup chopped green bell pepper
1/3 cup chopped yellow bell pepper
1/3 cup finely chopped green onions
½ cup orange juice
½ cup fresh lime juice
¼ tsp. dry mustard
¼ tsp. ground red pepper
2 garlic cloves, crushed
½ cup chopped tomato

2 cups fresh or frozen black-eyed
    peas, cooked
2 tbsp. chopped pickled pepper-
    oncini peppers
1½ tsp. Cajun seasoning
1 lb. medium shrimp, peeled and de-
    veined
½ lb. sea scallops
1 tsp. vegetable oil
8 cups thinly sliced mustard greens
    or romaine lettuce

Cook bacon in a large nonstick skillet over medium-high heat until crisp. Remove bacon from skillet, crumble and set aside. Add celery, bell peppers and onions to bacon fat in skillet and sauté for 1 minute. Set aside. Combine orange juice, lime juice, mustard, red pepper and garlic in a large bowl and stir well. Add celery mixture, peas, tomato and pickled peppers and toss well. Cover and chill. Sprinkle Cajun seasoning over the shrimp and scallops. Heat oil in skillet over high heat. Add seafood and sauté for 3 minutes. Spoon seafood into a bowl, and then cover and chill. Place 2 cups of the greens in each of 4 salad bowls and top with 1 cup of the pea mixture. Arrange one-fourth of the seafood over each salad and sprinkle each with 1½ tsp bacon. Serves 4.

Nutritional Information: 333 calories; 7.1g fat (19% calories from fat); 38.2g protein; 31.3g carbohydrates; 3.3g fiber; 154g cholesterol; 733mg sodium

Asian Party Mix

2 cups crispy corn cereal squares
    (such as Corn Chex®)
2 cups crispy rice cereal squares
    (such as Rice Chex®)
2 cups sesame rice crackers, broken
1 cup tiny fat-free pretzel twists
¾ cup wasabi peas
3 tbsp. unsalted butter

¼ cup lightly salted dry-roasted
    peanuts
1 tbsp. sugar
1 tbsp. curry powder
1 tbsp. low-sodium soy sauce
1 tsp. Worcestershire sauce
½ tsp. garlic powder
½ tsp. ground cumin

¼ tsp. salt   nonstick cooking spray
¼ tsp. ground red pepper

Preheat oven to 200° F. Combine corn cereal, rice cereal, sesame rice crackers, pretzel twists, wasabi peas and peanuts in a large bowl and set aside. Melt the butter in a small saucepan over medium heat. Add sugar, curry powder, soy sauce, Worcestershire sauce, garlic powder, cumin, salt and red pepper and stir with a whisk. Pour butter mixture over cereal mixture, tossing gently to coat. Spread the mixture onto a jellyroll pan coated with nonstick cooking spray. Bake at 200° F for 45 minutes. Cool completely before serving. Serves 8 (½ cup serving size).

Nutritional Information: 116 calories; 3.7g fat (32% calories from fat); 2.9g protein; 18.6g carbohydrates; 1.2g fiber; 6mg cholesterol; 269mg sodium

Banana Breakfast Smoothie
½ cup 1% lowfat milk $1/_8$ tsp. ground nutmeg
½ cup crushed ice   1 frozen sliced ripe large banana
1 tbsp. honey   1 cup plain Greek 2% yogurt

Combine milk, ice, honey, nutmeg and banana in a blender and process for 2 minutes or until smooth. Add yogurt and process just until blended. Serve immediately. Serves 2 (1 cup serving size).

Nutritional Information: 212 calories; 3.6g fat (15% calories from fat); 14.2g protein; 34.2g carbohydrates; 2g fiber; 9mg cholesterol; 75mg sodium

Chili-Spiced Almonds
1 tbsp. water   1 tsp. paprika
1 large egg white   1 tsp. ground cumin
1 lb. almonds, raw and unblanched   1 tsp. ground coriander
½ cup sugar   ½ tsp. chili powder
1 tbsp. salt   nonstick cooking spray

Preheat oven to 300° F. Combine 1 tbsp. water and egg white in a large bowl, and then stir with a whisk until foamy. Add almonds and toss well to coat. Place the almonds in a colander and drain for 5 minutes. Combine almonds, sugar, salt, paprika, cumin, coriander and chili powder in a large bowl and toss to coat. Spread almond mixture in a single layer on a jellyroll pan coated with nonstick cooking spray. Bake at 300° F for 15 minutes. Stir the almond mixture and reduce the oven temperature to 275° F. Bake the mixture an additional 40 minutes, stirring every 10 minutes. Remove the almond mixture from the oven and cool for 5 minutes. Break apart any clusters. Cool completely. Store at room temperature in an airtight container for up to a week. Makes 4 cups (2 tbsp. serving size).

Nutritional Information: 98 calories; 7.2g fat (67% calories from fat); 3.1g protein; 6g carbohydrates; 1.8g fiber; 0mg cholesterol; 221mg sodium

Member Survey

Please answer the following questions to help your leader plan your First Place 4 Health meetings so that your needs might be met in this session. Give this form to your leader at the first group meeting.

Name _____   Birth date _____

Please list those who live in your household.

Name	Relationship	Age

What church do you attend? _____

Are you interested in receiving more information about our church?

    Yes   No

Occupation _____

What talent or area of expertise would you be willing to share with our class?

_____

Why did you join First Place 4 Health?

_____

With notice, would you be willing to lead a Bible study discussion one week?

    Yes   No

Are you comfortable praying out loud? _____

If the assistant leader were absent, would you be willing to assist in weighing in members and possibly evaluating the Live It Trackers?

    Yes   No

Any other comments:

_____
_____

Personal Weight and Measurement Record

Week	Weight	+ or -	Goal this Session	Pounds to goal
1				
2				
3				
4				
5				
6				
7				
8				
9				
10				
11				
12				

Beginning Measurements

Waist _____ Hips _____ Thighs _____ Chest _____

Ending Measurements

Waist _____ Hips _____ Thighs _____ Chest _____

First Place 4 Health
Prayer Partner

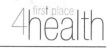

*But thanks be to God! He gives us the victory
through our Lord Jesus Christ.*

1 CORINTHIANS 15:57

Date: _____

Name: _____

Home Phone: (____) _____

Work Phone: (____) _____

Email: _____

Personal Prayer Concerns:

_____

_____

_____

_____

_____

_____

_____

This form is for prayer requests that are personal to you and your journey in First Place 4 Health. Please complete this form and have it ready to turn in when you arrive at your group meeting.

First Place 4 Health
Prayer Partner

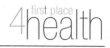

HEALTHY HOLIDAY
LIVING
Week
2

*Do not be anxious about anything, but in everything, by prayer and petition
with thanksgiving, present your requests to God.*

PHILIPPIANS 4:6

Date: _____

Name: _____

Home Phone: (_____) _____

Work Phone: (_____) _____

Email: _____

Personal Prayer Concerns:

_____

_____

_____

_____

_____

_____

This form is for prayer requests that are personal to you and your journey in First Place 4 Health. Please complete this form and have it ready to turn in when you arrive at your group meeting.

First Place 4 Health
Prayer Partner

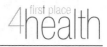

HEALTHY HOLIDAY
LIVING
Week
3

You will be with child and will give birth to a son,
and you are to give him the name Jesus.

LUKE 1:31

Date: _____

Name: _____

Home Phone: (_____) _____

Work Phone: (_____) _____

Email: _____

Personal Prayer Concerns:

_____

_____

_____

_____

_____

_____

_____

This form is for prayer requests that are personal to you and your journey in First Place 4 Health. Please complete this form and have it ready to turn in when you arrive at your group meeting.

First Place 4 Health
Prayer Partner

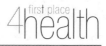

He will be great and will be called the Son of the Most High.
The Lord God will give him the throne of his father David.

LUKE 1:32

Date: _____

Name: _____

Home Phone: (_____) _____

Work Phone: (_____) _____

Email: _____

Personal Prayer Concerns:

_____

_____

_____

_____

_____

_____

_____

This form is for prayer requests that are personal to you and your journey in First Place 4 Health. Please complete this form and have it ready to turn in when you arrive at your group meeting.

First Place 4 Health
Prayer Partner

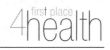

HEALTHY HOLIDAY
LIVING
Week
5

He put a new song in my mouth, a hymn of praise to our God.

PSALM 40:3

Date: _____

Name: _____

Home Phone: (____) _____

Work Phone: (____) _____

Email: _____

Personal Prayer Concerns:

_____

_____

_____

_____

_____

_____

_____

This form is for prayer requests that are personal to you and your journey in First Place 4 Health. Please complete this form and have it ready to turn in when you arrive at your group meeting.

First Place 4 Health
Prayer Partner

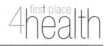

HEALTHY HOLIDAY
LIVING
Week
6

Yet I am writing you a new command; its truth is seen in him and you,
because the darkness is passing and the true light is already shining.

1 JOHN 2:8

Date: _____

Name: _____

Home Phone: (_____) _____

Work Phone: (_____) _____

Email: _____

Personal Prayer Concerns:

_____

_____

_____

_____

_____

_____

_____

This form is for prayer requests that are personal to you and your journey in First Place 4 Health. Please complete this form and have it ready to turn in when you arrive at your group meeting.

Live It Tracker

Name: _____ Loss/gain: _____ lbs.

Date: _____ Week #: _____ Calorie Range: _____ My food goal for next week: _____

Activity Level: None, < 30 min/day, 30-60 min/day, 60+ min/day My activity goal for next week: _____

Group	Daily Calories							
	1300-1400	1500-1600	1700-1800	1900-2000	2100-2200	2300-2400	2500-2600	2700-2800
Fruits	1.5-2 c.	1.5-2 c.	1.5-2 c.	2-2.5 c.	2-2.5 c.	2.5-3.5 c.	3.5-4.5 c.	3.5-4.5 c.
Vegetables	1.5-2 c.	2-2.5 c.	2.5-3 c.	2.5-3 c.	3-3.5 c.	3.5-4.5 c.	4.5-5 c.	4.5-5 c.
Grains	5 oz-eq.	5-6 oz-eq.	6-7 oz-eq.	6-7 oz-eq.	7-8 oz-eq.	8-9 oz-eq.	9-10 oz-eq.	10-11 oz-eq.
Meat & Beans	4 oz-eq.	5 oz-eq.	5-5.5 oz-eq.	5.5-6.5 oz-eq.	6.5-7 oz-eq.	7-7.5 oz-eq.	7-7.5 oz-eq.	7.5-8 oz-eq.
Milk	2-3 c.	3 c.	3 c.	3 c.	3 c.	3 c.	3 c.	3 c.
Healthy Oils	4 tsp.	5 tsp.	5 tsp.	6 tsp.	6 tsp.	7 tsp.	8 tsp.	8 tsp.

Breakfast: _____ Lunch: _____

Dinner: _____ Snack: _____

Group	Fruits	Vegetables	Grains	Meat & Beans	Milk	Oils
Goal Amount						
Estimate Your Total						
Increase ⇧ or Decrease? ⇩						

Physical Activity: _____ Spiritual Activity: _____

Steps/Miles/Minutes: _____

Breakfast: _____ Lunch: _____

Dinner: _____ Snack: _____

Group	Fruits	Vegetables	Grains	Meat & Beans	Milk	Oils
Goal Amount						
Estimate Your Total						
Increase ⇧ or Decrease? ⇩						

Physical Activity: _____ Spiritual Activity: _____

Steps/Miles/Minutes: _____

Breakfast: _____ Lunch: _____

Dinner: _____ Snack: _____

Group	Fruits	Vegetables	Grains	Meat & Beans	Milk	Oils
Goal Amount						
Estimate Your Total						
Increase ⇧ or Decrease? ⇩						

Physical Activity: _____ Spiritual Activity: _____

Steps/Miles/Minutes: _____

Day/Date:

Day/Date: _____

Breakfast: _____ _____ Lunch: _____

Dinner: _____ Snack: _____

Group	Fruits	Vegetables	Grains	Meat & Beans	Milk	Oils
Goal Amount						
Estimate Your Total						
Increase ⬆ or Decrease? ⬇						

Physical Activity: _____ Spiritual Activity: _____

Steps/Miles/Minutes: _____ _____

Day/Date: _____

Breakfast: _____ Lunch: _____

Dinner: _____ Snack: _____

Group	Fruits	Vegetables	Grains	Meat & Beans	Milk	Oils
Goal Amount						
Estimate Your Total						
Increase ⬆ or Decrease? ⬇						

Physical Activity: _____ Spiritual Activity: _____

Steps/Miles/Minutes: _____ _____

Day/Date: _____

Breakfast: _____ Lunch: _____

Dinner: _____ Snack: _____

Group	Fruits	Vegetables	Grains	Meat & Beans	Milk	Oils
Goal Amount						
Estimate Your Total						
Increase ⬆ or Decrease? ⬇						

Physical Activity: _____ Spiritual Activity: _____

Steps/Miles/Minutes: _____ _____

Day/Date: _____

Breakfast: _____ Lunch: _____

Dinner: _____ Snack: _____

Group	Fruits	Vegetables	Grains	Meat & Beans	Milk	Oils
Goal Amount						
Estimate Your Total						
Increase ⬆ or Decrease? ⬇						

Physical Activity: _____ Spiritual Activity: _____

Steps/Miles/Minutes: _____ _____

Live It Tracker

Name: _____ Loss/gain: _____ lbs.

Date: _____ Week #: _____ Calorie Range: _____ My food goal for next week: _____

Activity Level: None, < 30 min/day, 30-60 min/day, 60+ min/day My activity goal for next week: _____

Group	Daily Calories							
	1300-1400	1500-1600	1700-1800	1900-2000	2100-2200	2300-2400	2500-2600	2700-2800
Fruits	1.5-2 c.	1.5-2 c.	1.5-2 c.	2-2.5 c.	2-2.5 c.	2.5-3.5 c.	3.5-4.5 c.	3.5-4.5 c.
Vegetables	1.5-2 c.	2-2.5 c.	2.5-3 c.	2.5-3 c.	3-3.5 c.	3.5-4.5 c.	4.5-5 c.	4.5-5 c.
Grains	5 oz-eq.	5-6 oz-eq.	6-7 oz-eq.	6-7 oz-eq.	7-8 oz-eq.	8-9 oz-eq.	9-10 oz-eq.	10-11 oz-eq.
Meat & Beans	4 oz-eq.	5 oz-eq.	5-5.5 oz-eq.	5.5-6.5 oz-eq.	6.5-7 oz-eq.	7-7.5 oz-eq.	7-7.5 oz-eq.	7.5-8 oz-eq.
Milk	2-3 c.	3 c.	3 c.	3 c.	3 c.	3 c.	3 c.	3 c.
Healthy Oils	4 tsp.	5 tsp.	5 tsp.	6 tsp.	6 tsp.	7 tsp.	8 tsp.	8 tsp.

Day/Date:

Breakfast: _____ Lunch: _____

Dinner: _____ Snack: _____

Group	Fruits	Vegetables	Grains	Meat & Beans	Milk	Oils
Goal Amount						
Estimate Your Total						
Increase ⇧ or Decrease? ⇩						

Physical Activity: _____ Spiritual Activity: _____

Steps/Miles/Minutes: _____

Day/Date:

Breakfast: _____ Lunch: _____

Dinner: _____ Snack: _____

Group	Fruits	Vegetables	Grains	Meat & Beans	Milk	Oils
Goal Amount						
Estimate Your Total						
Increase ⇧ or Decrease? ⇩						

Physical Activity: _____ Spiritual Activity: _____

Steps/Miles/Minutes: _____

Day/Date:

Breakfast: _____ Lunch: _____

Dinner: _____ Snack: _____

Group	Fruits	Vegetables	Grains	Meat & Beans	Milk	Oils
Goal Amount						
Estimate Your Total						
Increase ⇧ or Decrease? ⇩						

Physical Activity: _____ Spiritual Activity: _____

Steps/Miles/Minutes: _____

Day/Date: _____

Breakfast: _____   Lunch: _____

Dinner: _____   Snack: _____

Group	Fruits	Vegetables	Grains	Meat & Beans	Milk	Oils
Goal Amount						
Estimate Your Total						
Increase ⇧ or Decrease? ⇩						

Physical Activity: _____   Spiritual Activity: _____

Steps/Miles/Minutes: _____

Day/Date: _____

Breakfast: _____   Lunch: _____

Dinner: _____   Snack: _____

Group	Fruits	Vegetables	Grains	Meat & Beans	Milk	Oils
Goal Amount						
Estimate Your Total						
Increase ⇧ or Decrease? ⇩						

Physical Activity: _____   Spiritual Activity: _____

Steps/Miles/Minutes: _____

Day/Date: _____

Breakfast: _____   Lunch: _____

Dinner: _____   Snack: _____

Group	Fruits	Vegetables	Grains	Meat & Beans	Milk	Oils
Goal Amount						
Estimate Your Total						
Increase ⇧ or Decrease? ⇩						

Physical Activity: _____   Spiritual Activity: _____

Steps/Miles/Minutes: _____

Day/Date: _____

Breakfast: _____   Lunch: _____

Dinner: _____   Snack: _____

Group	Fruits	Vegetables	Grains	Meat & Beans	Milk	Oils
Goal Amount						
Estimate Your Total						
Increase ⇧ or Decrease? ⇩						

Physical Activity: _____   Spiritual Activity: _____

Steps/Miles/Minutes: _____

Live It Tracker

Name: _____ Loss/gain: _____ lbs.

Date: _____ Week #: _____ Calorie Range: _____ My food goal for next week: _____

Activity Level: None, < 30 min/day, 30-60 min/day, 60+ min/day My activity goal for next week: _____

Group	Daily Calories							
	1300-1400	1500-1600	1700-1800	1900-2000	2100-2200	2300-2400	2500-2600	2700-2800
Fruits	1.5-2 c.	1.5-2 c.	1.5-2 c.	2-2.5 c.	2-2.5 c.	2.5-3.5 c.	3.5-4.5 c.	3.5-4.5 c.
Vegetables	1.5-2 c.	2-2.5 c.	2.5-3 c.	2.5-3 c.	3-3.5 c.	3.5-4.5 c.	4.5-5 c.	4.5-5 c.
Grains	5 oz-eq.	5-6 oz-eq.	6-7 oz-eq.	6-7 oz-eq.	7-8 oz-eq.	8-9 oz-eq.	9-10 oz-eq.	10-11 oz-eq.
Meat & Beans	4 oz-eq.	5 oz-eq.	5-5.5 oz-eq.	5.5-6.5 oz-eq.	6.5-7 oz-eq.	7-7.5 oz-eq.	7-7.5 oz-eq.	7.5-8 oz-eq.
Milk	2-3 c.	3 c.	3 c.	3 c.	3 c.	3 c.	3 c.	3 c.
Healthy Oils	4 tsp.	5 tsp.	5 tsp.	6 tsp.	6 tsp.	7 tsp.	8 tsp.	8 tsp.

Day/Date:

Breakfast: _____   Lunch: _____

Dinner: _____   Snack: _____

Group	Fruits	Vegetables	Grains	Meat & Beans	Milk	Oils
Goal Amount						
Estimate Your Total						
Increase ⬆ or Decrease? ⬇						

Physical Activity: _____   Spiritual Activity: _____

Steps/Miles/Minutes: _____

Day/Date:

Breakfast: _____   Lunch: _____

Dinner: _____   Snack: _____

Group	Fruits	Vegetables	Grains	Meat & Beans	Milk	Oils
Goal Amount						
Estimate Your Total						
Increase ⬆ or Decrease? ⬇						

Physical Activity: _____   Spiritual Activity: _____

Steps/Miles/Minutes: _____

Day/Date:

Breakfast: _____   Lunch: _____

Dinner: _____   Snack: _____

Group	Fruits	Vegetables	Grains	Meat & Beans	Milk	Oils
Goal Amount						
Estimate Your Total						
Increase ⬆ or Decrease? ⬇						

Physical Activity: _____   Spiritual Activity: _____

Steps/Miles/Minutes: _____

Day/Date: _____

Breakfast: _____ Lunch: _____

Dinner: _____ Snack: _____

Group	Fruits	Vegetables	Grains	Meat & Beans	Milk	Oils
Goal Amount						
Estimate Your Total						
Increase ⬆ or Decrease? ⬇						

Physical Activity: _____ Spiritual Activity: _____

Steps/Miles/Minutes: _____ _____

Day/Date: _____

Breakfast: _____ Lunch: _____

Dinner: _____ Snack: _____

Group	Fruits	Vegetables	Grains	Meat & Beans	Milk	Oils
Goal Amount						
Estimate Your Total						
Increase ⬆ or Decrease? ⬇						

Physical Activity: _____ Spiritual Activity: _____

Steps/Miles/Minutes: _____ _____

Day/Date: _____

Breakfast: _____ Lunch: _____

Dinner: _____ Snack: _____

Group	Fruits	Vegetables	Grains	Meat & Beans	Milk	Oils
Goal Amount						
Estimate Your Total						
Increase ⬆ or Decrease? ⬇						

Physical Activity: _____ Spiritual Activity: _____

Steps/Miles/Minutes: _____ _____

Day/Date: _____

Breakfast: _____ Lunch: _____

Dinner: _____ Snack: _____

Group	Fruits	Vegetables	Grains	Meat & Beans	Milk	Oils
Goal Amount						
Estimate Your Total						
Increase ⬆ or Decrease? ⬇						

Physical Activity: _____ Spiritual Activity: _____

Steps/Miles/Minutes: _____ _____

Live It Tracker

Name: _____ Loss/gain: _____ lbs.

Date: _____ Week #: _____ Calorie Range: _____ My food goal for next week: _____

Activity Level: None, < 30 min/day, 30-60 min/day, 60+ min/day My activity goal for next week: _____

Group	Daily Calories							
	1300-1400	1500-1600	1700-1800	1900-2000	2100-2200	2300-2400	2500-2600	2700-2800
Fruits	1.5-2 c.	1.5-2 c.	1.5-2 c.	2-2.5 c.	2-2.5 c.	2.5-3.5 c.	3.5-4.5 c.	3.5-4.5 c.
Vegetables	1.5-2 c.	2-2.5 c.	2.5-3 c.	2.5-3 c.	3-3.5 c.	3.5-4.5 c.	4.5-5 c.	4.5-5 c.
Grains	5 oz-eq.	5-6 oz-eq.	6-7 oz-eq.	6-7 oz-eq.	7-8 oz-eq.	8-9 oz-eq.	9-10 oz-eq.	10-11 oz-eq.
Meat & Beans	4 oz-eq.	5 oz-eq.	5-5.5 oz-eq.	5.5-6.5 oz-eq.	6.5-7 oz-eq.	7-7.5 oz-eq.	7-7.5 oz-eq.	7.5-8 oz-eq.
Milk	2-3 c.	3 c.	3 c.	3 c.	3 c.	3 c.	3 c.	3 c.
Healthy Oils	4 tsp.	5 tsp.	5 tsp.	6 tsp.	6 tsp.	7 tsp.	8 tsp.	8 tsp.

Day/Date:

Breakfast: _____ Lunch: _____

Dinner: _____ Snack: _____

Group	Fruits	Vegetables	Grains	Meat & Beans	Milk	Oils
Goal Amount						
Estimate Your Total						
Increase ⇧ or Decrease? ⇩						

Physical Activity: _____ Spiritual Activity: _____

Steps/Miles/Minutes: _____

Day/Date:

Breakfast: _____ Lunch: _____

Dinner: _____ Snack: _____

Group	Fruits	Vegetables	Grains	Meat & Beans	Milk	Oils
Goal Amount						
Estimate Your Total						
Increase ⇧ or Decrease? ⇩						

Physical Activity: _____ Spiritual Activity: _____

Steps/Miles/Minutes: _____

Day/Date:

Breakfast: _____ Lunch: _____

Dinner: _____ Snack: _____

Group	Fruits	Vegetables	Grains	Meat & Beans	Milk	Oils
Goal Amount						
Estimate Your Total						
Increase ⇧ or Decrease? ⇩						

Physical Activity: _____ Spiritual Activity: _____

Steps/Miles/Minutes: _____

Day/Date:

Breakfast: _____ Lunch: _____

Dinner: _____ Snack: _____

Group	Fruits	Vegetables	Grains	Meat & Beans	Milk	Oils
Goal Amount						
Estimate Your Total						
Increase ⇧ or Decrease? ⇩						

Physical Activity: _____ Spiritual Activity: _____

Steps/Miles/Minutes: _____ _____

Day/Date:

Breakfast: _____ Lunch: _____

Dinner: _____ Snack: _____

Group	Fruits	Vegetables	Grains	Meat & Beans	Milk	Oils
Goal Amount						
Estimate Your Total						
Increase ⇧ or Decrease? ⇩						

Physical Activity: _____ Spiritual Activity: _____

Steps/Miles/Minutes: _____ _____

Day/Date:

Breakfast: _____ Lunch: _____

Dinner: _____ Snack: _____

Group	Fruits	Vegetables	Grains	Meat & Beans	Milk	Oils
Goal Amount						
Estimate Your Total						
Increase ⇧ or Decrease? ⇩						

Physical Activity: _____ Spiritual Activity: _____

Steps/Miles/Minutes: _____ _____

Day/Date:

Breakfast: _____ Lunch: _____

Dinner: _____ Snack: _____

Group	Fruits	Vegetables	Grains	Meat & Beans	Milk	Oils
Goal Amount						
Estimate Your Total						
Increase ⇧ or Decrease? ⇩						

Physical Activity: _____ Spiritual Activity: _____

Steps/Miles/Minutes: _____ _____

Live It Tracker

Name: _____ Loss/gain: _____ lbs.

Date: _____ Week #: _____ Calorie Range: _____ My food goal for next week: _____

Activity Level: None, < 30 min/day, 30-60 min/day, 60+ min/day My activity goal for next week: _____

Group	Daily Calories							
	1300-1400	1500-1600	1700-1800	1900-2000	2100-2200	2300-2400	2500-2600	2700-2800
Fruits	1.5-2 c.	1.5-2 c.	1.5-2 c.	2-2.5 c.	2-2.5 c.	2.5-3.5 c.	3.5-4.5 c.	3.5-4.5 c.
Vegetables	1.5-2 c.	2-2.5 c.	2.5-3 c.	2.5-3 c.	3-3.5 c.	3.5-4.5 c.	4.5-5 c.	4.5-5 c.
Grains	5 oz-eq.	5-6 oz-eq.	6-7 oz-eq.	6-7 oz-eq.	7-8 oz-eq.	8-9 oz-eq.	9-10 oz-eq.	10-11 oz-eq.
Meat & Beans	4 oz-eq.	5 oz-eq.	5-5.5 oz-eq.	5.5-6.5 oz-eq.	6.5-7 oz-eq.	7-7.5 oz-eq.	7-7.5 oz-eq.	7.5-8 oz-eq.
Milk	2-3 c.	3 c.	3 c.	3 c.	3 c.	3 c.	3 c.	3 c.
Healthy Oils	4 tsp.	5 tsp.	5 tsp.	6 tsp.	6 tsp.	7 tsp.	8 tsp.	8 tsp.

Day/Date: _____

Breakfast: _____ Lunch: _____

Dinner: _____ Snack: _____

Group	Fruits	Vegetables	Grains	Meat & Beans	Milk	Oils
Goal Amount						
Estimate Your Total						
Increase ⇧ or Decrease? ⇩						

Physical Activity: _____ Spiritual Activity: _____

Steps/Miles/Minutes: _____

Day/Date: _____

Breakfast: _____ Lunch: _____

Dinner: _____ Snack: _____

Group	Fruits	Vegetables	Grains	Meat & Beans	Milk	Oils
Goal Amount						
Estimate Your Total						
Increase ⇧ or Decrease? ⇩						

Physical Activity: _____ Spiritual Activity: _____

Steps/Miles/Minutes: _____

Day/Date: _____

Breakfast: _____ Lunch: _____

Dinner: _____ Snack: _____

Group	Fruits	Vegetables	Grains	Meat & Beans	Milk	Oils
Goal Amount						
Estimate Your Total						
Increase ⇧ or Decrease? ⇩						

Physical Activity: _____ Spiritual Activity: _____

Steps/Miles/Minutes: _____

Day/Date: ___

Breakfast: _____   Lunch: _____
_____   _____
Dinner: _____   Snack: _____
_____   _____

Group	Fruits	Vegetables	Grains	Meat & Beans	Milk	Oils
Goal Amount						
Estimate Your Total						
Increase ⇧ or Decrease? ⇩						

Physical Activity: _____   Spiritual Activity: _____
Steps/Miles/Minutes: _____ _____

Day/Date: ___

Breakfast: _____   Lunch: _____
_____   _____
Dinner: _____   Snack: _____
_____   _____

Group	Fruits	Vegetables	Grains	Meat & Beans	Milk	Oils
Goal Amount						
Estimate Your Total						
Increase ⇧ or Decrease? ⇩						

Physical Activity: _____   Spiritual Activity: _____
Steps/Miles/Minutes: _____ _____

Day/Date: ___

Breakfast: _____   Lunch: _____
_____   _____
Dinner: _____   Snack: _____
_____   _____

Group	Fruits	Vegetables	Grains	Meat & Beans	Milk	Oils
Goal Amount						
Estimate Your Total						
Increase ⇧ or Decrease? ⇩						

Physical Activity: _____   Spiritual Activity: _____
Steps/Miles/Minutes: _____ _____

Day/Date: ___

Breakfast: _____   Lunch: _____
_____   _____
Dinner: _____   Snack: _____
_____   _____

Group	Fruits	Vegetables	Grains	Meat & Beans	Milk	Oils
Goal Amount						
Estimate Your Total						
Increase ⇧ or Decrease? ⇩						

Physical Activity: _____   Spiritual Activity: _____
Steps/Miles/Minutes: _____ _____

Live It Tracker

Name: _____   Loss/gain: _____ lbs.

Date: _____ Week #: _____ Calorie Range: _____ My food goal for next week: _____

Activity Level: None, < 30 min/day, 30-60 min/day, 60+ min/day   My activity goal for next week: _____

Group	Daily Calories							
	1300-1400	1500-1600	1700-1800	1900-2000	2100-2200	2300-2400	2500-2600	2700-2800
Fruits	1.5-2 c.	1.5-2 c.	1.5-2 c.	2-2.5 c.	2-2.5 c.	2.5-3.5 c.	3.5-4.5 c.	3.5-4.5 c.
Vegetables	1.5-2 c.	2-2.5 c.	2.5-3 c.	2.5-3 c.	3-3.5 c.	3.5-4.5 c.	4.5-5 c.	4.5-5 c.
Grains	5 oz-eq.	5-6 oz-eq.	6-7 oz-eq.	6-7 oz-eq.	7-8 oz-eq.	8-9 oz-eq.	9-10 oz-eq.	10-11 oz-eq.
Meat & Beans	4 oz-eq.	5 oz-eq.	5-5.5 oz-eq.	5.5-6.5 oz-eq.	6.5-7 oz-eq.	7-7.5 oz-eq.	7-7.5 oz-eq.	7.5-8 oz-eq.
Milk	2-3 c.	3 c.	3 c.	3 c.	3 c.	3 c.	3 c.	3 c.
Healthy Oils	4 tsp.	5 tsp.	5 tsp.	6 tsp.	6 tsp.	7 tsp.	8 tsp.	8 tsp.

Day/Date: _____

Breakfast: _____   Lunch: _____

Dinner: _____   Snack: _____

Group	Fruits	Vegetables	Grains	Meat & Beans	Milk	Oils
Goal Amount						
Estimate Your Total						
Increase ⇧ or Decrease? ⇩						

Physical Activity: _____   Spiritual Activity: _____

Steps/Miles/Minutes: _____

Day/Date: _____

Breakfast: _____   Lunch: _____

Dinner: _____   Snack: _____

Group	Fruits	Vegetables	Grains	Meat & Beans	Milk	Oils
Goal Amount						
Estimate Your Total						
Increase ⇧ or Decrease? ⇩						

Physical Activity: _____   Spiritual Activity: _____

Steps/Miles/Minutes: _____

Day/Date: _____

Breakfast: _____   Lunch: _____

Dinner: _____   Snack: _____

Group	Fruits	Vegetables	Grains	Meat & Beans	Milk	Oils
Goal Amount						
Estimate Your Total						
Increase ⇧ or Decrease? ⇩						

Physical Activity: _____   Spiritual Activity: _____

Steps/Miles/Minutes: _____

Day/Date: _____

Breakfast: _____ Lunch: _____

Dinner: _____ Snack: _____

Group	Fruits	Vegetables	Grains	Meat & Beans	Milk	Oils
Goal Amount						
Estimate Your Total						
Increase ⬆ or Decrease? ⬇						

Physical Activity: _____ Spiritual Activity: _____

Steps/Miles/Minutes: _____

Day/Date: _____

Breakfast: _____ Lunch: _____

Dinner: _____ Snack: _____

Group	Fruits	Vegetables	Grains	Meat & Beans	Milk	Oils
Goal Amount						
Estimate Your Total						
Increase ⬆ or Decrease? ⬇						

Physical Activity: _____ Spiritual Activity: _____

Steps/Miles/Minutes: _____

Day/Date: _____

Breakfast: _____ Lunch: _____

Dinner: _____ Snack: _____

Group	Fruits	Vegetables	Grains	Meat & Beans	Milk	Oils
Goal Amount						
Estimate Your Total						
Increase ⬆ or Decrease? ⬇						

Physical Activity: _____ Spiritual Activity: _____

Steps/Miles/Minutes: _____

Day/Date: _____

Breakfast: _____ Lunch: _____

Dinner: _____ Snack: _____

Group	Fruits	Vegetables	Grains	Meat & Beans	Milk	Oils
Goal Amount						
Estimate Your Total						
Increase ⬆ or Decrease? ⬇						

Physical Activity: _____ Spiritual Activity: _____

Steps/Miles/Minutes: _____

contributors

P.J. Bahr
Rapid City,
South Dakota

Luanne Blackburn
Indianapolis, Indiana

June Chapko
San Antonio, Texas

Kathlee Coleman
Santa Clarita, California

Charlotte Davis
Pangburn, Arizona

Delilah Dirksen
Greenland, New Hampshire

Vicki Heath
North Charleston, Edisto Island
South Carolina

Jean Krogh
Kewaunee, Wisconsin

Carole Lewis
Houston, Texas

Lisa Lewis
Spring Valley, Texas

Barbara Lukies
Farmborough Heights,
NSW, Australia

Judy Marshall
Gilmer, Texas

Sherry Mazza
Bayville, New Jersey

Paulette McDonald
Madisonville, Louisiana

Betha Jean McGee
Wall, Texas

Sarah Mielke
Louisville, Kentucky

Martha Rogers
Houston, Texas

Bev Schwind
Fairfield Glade, Tennessee

David Self
Houston, Texas

Karrie Smyth
Brandon, Manitoba, Canada

Carol Van Atta
Troutdale, Oregon

What Can God Do in Your Life in a Year?

Give God a Year Kit

The *Give God a Year* Kit contains everything you need to set aside one year and watch God's power change you from the inside out. Change will happen over the course of 12 months, but the right changes only happen when you set goals and take the right steps to achieve them. You will dream big about the changes you have longed for your whole life and receive practical, biblical, step-by-step guidance for seeing those dreams made into reality. In a culture of "right now," a year may seem like an eternity. A year in the hands of God, however, means change that will last eternally. The kit includes the *Give God a Year* trade book, *Give God a Year* journal, *Give God a Year* 365-day tear-off calendar, *Give God a Year* refrigerator magnet, *Give God a Year* mug, and an audio CD with a special message from national First Place 4 Health director, Carole Lewis.

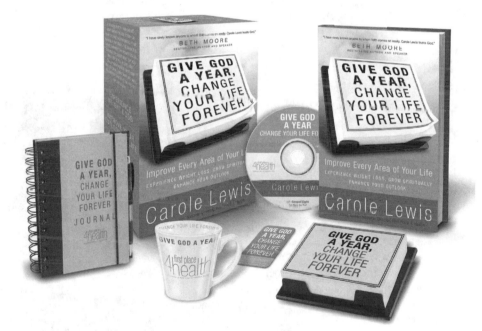

Give God a Year Kit
978.08307.52133 • $49.99
available at www.gospellight.com
and www.firstplace4health.com

Experience a First Place 4 Health Miracle

Teaching New Members Is Easy!

The First Place 4 Health Kit contains everything members need to live healthy, lose weight, make friends, and experience spiritual growth. With each resource, members will make positive changes in their thoughts and emotions, while transforming the way they fuel and recharge their bodies and relate to God.

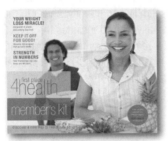

97808307.45890
$99.99 (A $145 Value!)

Member's Kit Contains:
- First Place 4 Health Hardcover Book
- Emotions & Eating DVD
- First Place 4 Health Member's Guide
- First Place 4 Health Prayer Journal
- Simple Ideas for Healthy Living
- First Place 4 Health Tote Bag
- Food on the Go Pocket Guide
- Why Should a Christian Be Physically Fit? DVD

I lost 74 pounds in 9 months!

**Abby Meloy,
New Life Christian Fellowship
Lake City, Florida**

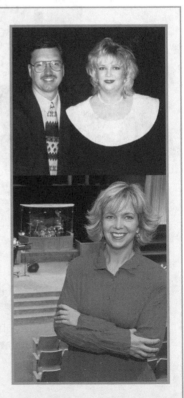

I am thankful for the First Place program. As a pastor's wife who remained at the 200-pound (+) mark for seven years, I can now say I am 135 pounds, a size 8, and I have maintained this weight.

In the beginning, I did not want to try First Place 4 Health. I did not want to weigh my food or take the time to learn the measurements, but the ladies in my church wanted the program, and I was a size 18/20, so I gave it a shot. After our first session, I was 27 pounds lighter and had new insights that my body is the temple of the Holy Spirit. It took me 9 months and 3 sessions to lose 74 pounds.

My new lifestyle has influenced my husband to lose 20 pounds and my 13-year-old daughter to lose 35 pounds. We are able to carry out the work of the ministry with much less fatigue. I now teach others in my church the First Place program and will be forever grateful that the Lord brought it into my life.

Influence Others to Put Christ First

Starting a Group Is Easy!

The First Place 4 Health Group Starter Kit includes everything you need to start and confidently lead your group into healthy living, weight loss, friendships, and spiritual growth. You will find lesson plans, training DVDs, a user-friendly food plan and other easy-to-use tools to help you lead members to a new way of thinking about health and Christ through a renewed mind, emotions, body and spirit.

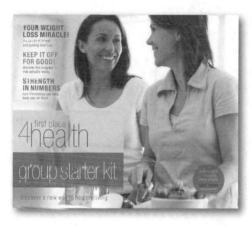

Group Starter Kit Contains:
- A Complete Member's Kit with Member Navigation Sheet
- First Place 4 Health Leader's Guide
- Begin with Christ Bible Study
- First Place 4 Health Orientation and Food Plan DVD
- How to Lead with Excellence DVD
- 25 Brochures on the First Place 4 Health Program

978.08307.45906
$199.99 (A $256 value!)

first place
4health
discover a new way to healthy living

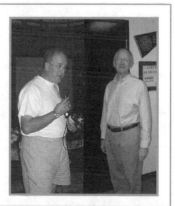

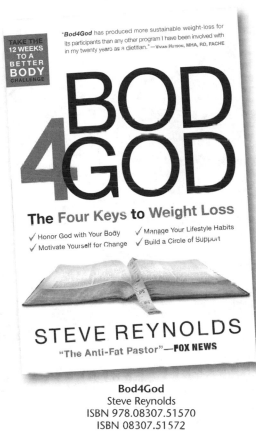
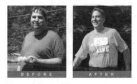